M000287224

Essentials of
Community-based Research

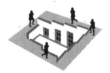

Qualitative Essentials

Series Editor: Janice Morse
University of Utah

Series Editorial Board: H. Russell Bernard, Kathy Charmaz, D. Jean Clandinin, Juliet Corbin, Carmen de la Cuesta, John Engel, Sue E. Estroff, Jane Gilgun, Jeffrey C. Johnson, Carl Mitcham, Katja Mruck, Judith Preissle, Jean J. Schensul, Sally Thorne, John van Maanen, Max van Manen

Qualitative Essentials is a book series providing a comprehensive but succinct overview of topics in qualitative inquiry. These books will fill an important niche in qualitative methods for students—and others new to the qualitative research—who require rapid but complete perspective on specific methods, strategies, and important topics. Written by leaders in qualitative inquiry, alone or in combination, these books will be an excellent resource for instructors and students from all disciplines. Proposals for the series should be sent to the series editor at explore@lcoastpress.com.

Titles in this series:
1. *Naturalistic Observation*, Michael V. Angrosino
2. *Essentials of Qualitative Inquiry*, Maria J. Mayan
3. *Essentials of Field Relationships*, Amy Kaler and Melanie A. Beres
4. *Essentials of Accessible Grounded Theory*, Phyllis Norerager Stern and Caroline Jane Porr
5. *Essentials of Qualitative Interviewing*, Karin Olson
6. *Essentials of Transdisciplinary Research*, Patricia Leavy
8. *Essentials of a Qualitative Doctorate*, Immy Holloway and Lorraine Brown
9. *Focus Group Research*, Martha Ann Carey and Jo-Ellen Asbury
10. *Essentials of Thinking Ethically in Qualitative Research*, Will C. van den Hoonaard and Deborah K. van den Hoonaard
11. *Essentials of Community-based Research*, Vera Caine and Judy Mill
12. *Essentials of Publishing Qualitative Research*, Mitchell Allen
13. *Essentials of Dyadic Interviewing*, David L. Morgan

Essentials of
Community-based Research

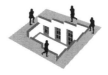

Vera Caine and Judy Mill

with contributions by Randy Jackson and Renée Masching

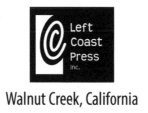

Walnut Creek, California

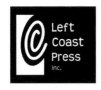

LEFT COAST PRESS, INC.
1630 North Main Street, #400
Walnut Creek, CA 94596
www.LCoastPress.com

Copyright © 2016 by Left Coast Press, Inc.

All rights reserved. No part of this publication may be reproduced, stored in a retrieval system, or transmitted in any form or by any means, electronic, mechanical, photo-copying, recording, or otherwise, without the prior permission of the publisher.

ISBN 978-1-62958-110-1 hardback
ISBN 978-1-62958-111-8 paperback
ISBN 978-1-62958-113-2 consumer eBook

Library of Congress Cataloging-in-Publication Data:

Caine, Vera.
Essentials of community-based research / Vera Caine and Judy Mill ; with contributions by Randy Jackson and Renee Masching.
    pages cm. — (Qualitative essentials ; 11)
  Includes bibliographical references and index.
    ISBN 978-1-62958-110-1 (hardback) — ISBN 978-1-62958-111-8 (paperback) — ISBN 978-1-62958-113-2 (consumer eBook)
    1. Community-based social service–Research–Methodology. 2. Community health services–Research–Methodology. 3. Community life–Research–Methodology. 4. Social sciences–Methodology. I. Mill, Judy, 1950- II. Title.
  HV11.C246 2015
  361.0072—dc23
                        2015028899

Printed in the United States of America

♾™ The paper used in this publication meets the minimum requirements of American National Standard for Information Sciences—Permanence of Paper for Printed Library Materials, ANSI/NISO Z39.48–1992.

Contents

Preface

I t was about two years ago that we sat with David[1] at the kitchen table
at his temporary home, only days before he passed away in 2013 after a
long and often difficult journey living with HIV. There are two things we
remember clearly about our visit: one was the far too baggy pair of long
coveralls David wore that day, coveralls that gave away his rapid weight
loss and deteriorating condition, but perhaps the more striking thing was
his continuous passion for community-based research. Both Judy and Vera
had known David for many years: he had been part of a project on HIV and
stigma together with Judy, and Vera had come to know him through our
most recent work on an HIV mentorship project for nurses. Both projects
were community-based research projects and involved people living with
HIV, community organizations, people living within communities affected
by HIV, and academics. David was an integral part of the projects, and
often the most critical voice. That day at the kitchen table, David talked
about upgrading his current computer equipment so that he could be
better connected and have more reliable Internet access. Over the previous
few months his deteriorating condition had made it difficult to visit places
within the community, including our offices at the university.

Starting this book by calling forth memories of David is important to
us. In many ways this book is a way for us to acknowledge those who have
shaped our lives and how we came to know and continued to learn about
community-based research. Yet, perhaps more important, it is David's passion that continues to hold us accountable to the research we are engaged
in. Vera remembers how David evoked both a deep sadness in her and a
smile by his active resistance to rules he felt were arbitrary, unjust, or just
simply didn't make sense; he never took "no" for an answer, particularly
when others relied on policies as a way to respond to his needs or concerns.
His resistance was often accompanied by a vigorous impatience; this too
became visible in his involvement with research projects. He often asked
us why our research took so long to shift care practices, policies, or attitudes of those around him. There were long e-mails, detailed telephone

messages, and meeting notes, all of which spoke about his wish to be part of larger and more systemic changes within the communities where he lived. For David, his involvement in research and teachings within university classrooms was about being part of changes to address issues of equity and social justice. Many experiences within his own life had placed him on the margins.

Our experiences in community-based research are primarily situated within the field of HIV. Many others have worked in diverse areas that are initiated by or of interest to the community. While HIV calls forth certain vulnerabilities and issues that may not be as present in other community-based research projects, we hope that some of our learnings and observations that we make visible in this book will resonate. David was a community activist for many years, and we fondly recall his writing in local papers and blogs. He saw himself as someone who wanted and could deeply shape the frontline work of HIV care and also the experiences of people living with HIV. The question he always posed to us still remains present as we think about and with community-based research: "What are you waiting for?"

David helped us understand community-based research from a place of experience, a place where we are called to live up to the principles and commitments to communities in which we are invested in and/or are a part of. There is an ever-increasing number of theoretical and research-based publications on community-based research, community-based participatory research, and community engagement, all of which offer great insights and trace important historical, ontological, and epistemological underpinnings. Yet for us, it is David who challenged us to think about our work, its impacts, and why it remains important for us as researchers to be grounded in the community. We hope that perhaps this book is a beginning for others to understand the complexities, possibilities, and challenges in community-based research and to answer David's question: "What are you waiting for?"

Plan of the Book

We have structured the book in four sections. In the first section, we provide an introduction to community-based research and draw attention to its key principles. Building on this understanding, in the second section of the book we provide details of two distinctively different studies to show what community-based research looks like in the field. One of the chapters in this section focuses on some frequently encountered design issues. We too focus on the development of more formal principles for research collaboration, which reflect one way of attending to the important aspects of working with multiple partners who have different stakes in the research. Given that multiple partners are involved in the research, we have included a chapter that focuses on the development of principles for research collaboration. In the third section, the focus is on the contexts and challenges in community-based research. Three chapters in this section evolve around the following key challenges: raising ethical questions, considering capacity, and working with diverse population. In chapter 8, Randy Jackson and Renée Masching focus on their experiences of working with and in Aboriginal communities. The fourth and last section looks at issues of enacting social justice in community-based research and also a discussion on the ways forward.

Acknowledgments

We have learned much from the commitment and passion of community members and organization over the years and would like to acknowledge their efforts in teaching us. We thank the participants who joined us in our research journeys. We are indebted to Hiroko Yamane, Aparajita Pyakuryal, Jean Chaw-Kant, and Lauren Starko for their assistance throughout the writing of this book; Mitch Allen was fabulous to work with!

Many organizations contributed funding to projects. We would like to acknowledge Health Canada for funding the "Challenging Lifestyles: Aboriginal Men and Women Living with HIV" project. The Canadian Institutes for Health Research (CIHR) provided the funding for the research projects "The Influence of Stigma on Access to Health Services by Persons with HIV Illness," "The Diagnosis and Care of HIV Infection in Canadian Aboriginal Youth," and the "Clinical Mentorship for Nurses in HIV Care." The Program of Research, "Strengthening Nurses' Capacity for HIV Policy Development in sub-Saharan Africa and the Caribbean," was carried out with support from the Global Health Research Initiative (GHRI), a collaborative research funding partnership of the Canadian Institutes of Health Research, the Canadian International Development

Agency, Health Canada, the International Development Research Centre, and the Public Health Agency of Canada. The Délįnę Uranium Research project was funded by the Canadian federal government.

We particularly extend our thanks to CIHR for their continuous support through the HIV Community-Based Research Programs. Without their support, the diversity and learnings about community-based research in Canada, particularly in the field of HIV, would not be possible; the benefits of aligning funding with research approaches that benefit and are grounded in community has proven to be critical.

Section I
History and Current Practice

1. What Is Community-based Research?

Community-based research has several historical roots and is often seen as grounded in post-positivism endeavors of research. Some value it for its recognition of local knowledge and experience, while for others it is research that compromises rigor in scientific processes. The debates are complex and often make visible the different theoretical and ideological positions of researchers, community members, and activists. Perhaps for most, community-based research is an approach to research that explicitly critiques the ontological and epistemological rigidity attributed to positivism while drawing on critical theory, feminism, anti-colonialism, and constructivism paradigms.

Community-based research comprises different things for different people. A number of disagreements in the field both propel it forward and at other times fragment the understanding and importance of the work.

Essentials of Community-based Research by Vera Caine and Judy Mill, 13–21. © 2016 Left Coast Press, Inc. All rights reserved.

For some academics, community-based research is a connection between researchers and community organizations, while for community organizations, community-based research may be about conducting their own research with or without the support of academics (Trussler & Marchand, 2005). In this debate several issues become evident: first, community-based research must start with a clear definition; second, community-based research must build capacity to undertake research (by capacity building we mean that resources, infrastructure, skills, knowledge, and leadership are developed); and last, there is a need to engage in the process of community-based research authentically, ethically, and meaningfully.

Defining Community-based Research

The broadest definitions of community-based research include an understanding that the research is grounded in community, serves the interest of the community, and actively engages citizens. Community-based research is geared towards creating an environment for, or directly affecting, social change. We find the definition advocated by the Community Health Scholars Program of the WK Kellogg Foundation (Kellogg Foundation, 2015) useful. They define community-based participatory research as

> [a] collaborative approach to research that equitably involves all partners in the research process and recognizes the unique strengths that each brings. [Community-based participatory research] begins with a research topic of importance to the community and has the aim of combining knowledge with action and achieving social change to improve health outcomes and eliminate health disparities.

Using this definition, it is apparent that community-based research is not a methodology or a set of methods that can be used, but rather an approach to research. This approach not only advances understanding or knowledge, but also aims to make a practical difference in the world (Flicker, 2008). It is inherently political, not only in its intention, but also in the process of democratizing the processes of knowledge production. Given its primary emphasis on community involvement in knowledge production and understanding of particular phenomena, it is necessary to be specific about who makes up the community.

Who Is the Community? What Is Participation?

The word *community* is often overused and evokes feelings of belonging without carefully considering and accounting for the diversity that exists within and among communities. The etymology of the word dates back to the late fourteenth century and stems from the Latin word *communitas*, which brings forward a sense of fellowship, courtesy, and the common and public. The origins of the word connect community to relationships with those who share feelings for each other, but community is also seen concretely as a body of people (Communitas, 2001–2005).

Drawing on this early understanding of what community means, it is important to see that community refers to more than a place or a geographical location, but that it also speaks to a sense of shared experience, relationships, and the reality that communities have a sense of organizing themselves. Drevdahl (2002) points out that "understanding the workings of power is integral to knowing community more fully" (p. 11). Recognizing these power dynamics within community is important, as these dynamics not only shape who participates in all phases of the research, but the ways in which the knowledge may be taken up later.

As we think carefully about community, we can see that in our own lives we belong to communities that are not homogenous, and that we are part of multiple communities simultaneously. While the etymology of the word *community* indicates a sense of commonality and shared space, there is also a sense of uncertainty, flexibility, and change present in communities. This more complex understanding of community calls forth that "[p]articipation in a community-based research project is a dynamic phenomenon that must be negotiated among an evolving web of roles and relationships" (Chung & Lounsbury, 2006, p. 2129).

Defining the evolving roles and relationships within each community-based research project is an ongoing process, shaped in part by understandings of the reason for the involvement of community as well as a continuum of understanding of what participation means. The involvement of the community is influenced frequently by the purpose and the scope of the research, but researchers using community-based research must also consider the contextual factors that are key in the implementation phase of the research. Given the intent of community-based research to create an environment where policies and practices can be changed, it is important to engage in discussion with communities about their involvement in the interpretation and application of the research findings or outcomes.

The level of involvement or participation of communities reflect a continuum. Loewenson, Laurell, Hogstedt, D'Ambruoso, and Shroff's (2014) description of the continuum is shown here:

Degree of Community Engagement

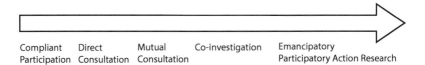

Compliant   Direct   Mutual   Co-investigation   Emancipatory
Participation   Consultation   Consultation   Participatory Action Research

Across the continuum, and regardless of the level of involvement of the community, in each research project it is important to reflect core elements of community-based research, including mutual respect and trust, capacity building, empowerment, and accountability and ownership (Cargo & Mercer, 2008).

Historical Roots

Community-based research is grounded historically in the work on action research by Kurt Lewin in the 1940s, as well as the work of Paulo Freire, Orlando Fals Borda, and feminist and postcolonial scholars around the world. For Kurt Lewin (1946), a German-American social psychologist, action research was a means to overcome social inequalities; he was particularly interested in problem solving and change. Kurt Lewin saw the importance of building strong partnerships between academics and communities and advocated a utilitarian approach that valued agreement and consensus. While participatory approaches also are concerned with problem solving and strong partnership approaches, "participatory research recognizes the challenges inherent in doing work where the powerful in society may resist when they feel their power threatened" (Flicker, Savan, McGrath, Kolenda, & Mildenberger, 2008a, p. 241). Paulo Freire (1973, 1989) emphasized much more emancipatory approaches and recognized issues of power and conflict.

Much of Paulo Freire's (1973, 1989) work was grounded in the strong belief that communities not only held knowledge, but that community members and organizations created knowledge. This shift in thinking validated

Encountering Scholars

Kurt Lewin (1890–1947) was a German-American social psychologist who made important contributions towards applied research, action research, and social processes. He is also considered a seminal theorist. His writing about action research is most important to community-based research. Toward the end of his life, he wrote about action research in relation to minority problems. For him, research leading to social action was critical and could be achieved through a series of steps that evolved much like a spiral (planning, action, fact-funding about the results/impact of the action).

Paulo Freire (1921–1997) was a Brazilian philosopher and an influential thinker on education. He contributed significantly to our understanding of critical pedagogy. His work focused on oppression and how education is linked to liberation and a sense of humanity. For Freire, education was a political act. He emphasized dialogue and the importance of working *with* people.

bell hooks (1952–) is an American feminist and social activist. She is particularly interested in race and gender and how these produce and perpetuate systems of oppression. In her early work she noted a lack of diversity within the feminist development of theory; she advocated that women and others should take note of differences. She also is instrumental in defining the development of intersectionality, pointing out that gender, class, and race are connected. hooks argues that loving communities are critical to move beyond issues, while she also works to address significant power structures that are embedded in classrooms or educational settings.

the importance of experience and emphasized that scholarship could no longer be considered neutral. Freire's thinking shaped community-based research in that it became clear that people must be actively involved in their learning and knowledge creation to address social justice concerns and to change their social-political conditions.

This foundation is later built upon by bell hooks, who states that the learning process must be reciprocal and mutual; for example, in research, the inquirer is also impacted and transformed along with the participants because the inquirer also participates, bringing her or his own narratives and interpretations into the relationship and the work. (Hunter et al., 2011, p. 49)

A strong link can also be traced between community-based research and the adult education movement in which political empowerment is connected to literacy and skill development (Hall, 1981, 1988) and knowledge creation is seen as an ideological process. At the same time, research grounded in and responsive to communities emerged through the work of oppressed communities in South America, Asia, and Africa in the 1970s (Minkler, 2005). In particular, since the 1970s, community-based research has been further developed as a result of the insistence of Indigenous peoples and organizations that represent them (Fletcher, 2003). The involvement of Indigenous peoples also brought with it a strong focus on the right to self-determination. As Cargo and Mercer (2008) have pointed out, self-determination has "emerged parallel to the sovereignty movements of indigenous people and the desire for other marginalized and underserved populations (e.g., HIV/AIDS and disability movements) to assert control over the research and programs that affect them" (p. 330).

As researchers and communities began to realize the potential inherent in community-based research to democratize knowledge, validate multiple sources of knowledge, and achieve change and self-determination, the demand for community-based research increased. During this time, through the popular education movement, research expanded to include/embrace/incorporate a focus on social and environmental justice, and to ensure that knowledge was translated into action. Marxist, queer, and feminist researchers further contributed to the development of community-based research, particularly by arguing for greater decision-making power over studies that took place within their communities.

Ontological and Epistemological Underpinnings

The historical foundations of community-based research already point to different ways of understanding not only *how we know* (epistemology), but also to how we might understand the *nature and relation of being* (ontology). Different ontological and epistemological understandings in turn also shape what tools researchers use and which methodologies are most appropriate. It is important to understand that community-based research is an approach to research and reflects both ontological and epistemological positions that are grounded in its historical development, but that diverse methodological choices (such as qualitative and quantitative designs) are possible within this approach.

Community-based research most often draws on constructivist and critical theoretical perspectives, as knowledge is socially created. Ultimately, community-based research "recognizes local knowledge systems as valid on their own epistemological foundations and views them as contributing to a larger understanding of the world and place of humans in it. It takes as an a priori assumption that research and science are not value free" (Fletcher, 2003, p. 32). Knowledge creation is transactional and interactive, reflecting participatory ways of being. Researchers and community members engage in interactive and highly reflective processes to develop practical knowledge that is relevant to the community. In this process, a focus on social change, as well as sustainability of relationships and interchanges, is key. Table 1.1 highlights the ontological, epistemological, and methodological distinctions among different paradigms.

Link to Inequities and Social Determinants of Health

Although the historical roots of community-based research have been well described, the development of this approach to research continues. This ongoing development is facilitated by learning from research initiated and conducted by community organizations as well as researchers continuing to seek possibilities to involve and work closely with communities during all phases of the research. More and more literature is now dedicated to examining completed research projects and exploring how relationships within and across communities can be widened and enhanced. The interest in community-based research continuous to grow, primarily because of a profound recognition that traditional approaches to research have failed to address increasing inequities and solve complex social and health disparities. This recognition is also mirrored in increasing obligations for researchers to engage in knowledge mobilization or knowledge translation efforts to show the merit and relevance of their research findings. This push does not come without an ongoing critique of applied social and health research, particularly when the creation of knowledge is not always predictable. The tension and power dynamics between academics, funding

Table 1.1   Philosophies of Science

	Positivism	Post-positivism	Critical Theory	Constructivism	Participatory
Ontology	There is a reality that can be observed. Truth can be discovered.	*Critical realism:* Reality exists, but we cannot have any objective or certain knowledge. Knowledge is incomplete.	*Historical realism:* History and power shape the reality of people's lives.	*Relativism:* Realities are constructed and situated in specific social contexts.	*Participative reality:* Reality can be understood through the experiences of people in relation. Mindfulness is essential.
Epistemology	*Objectivist:* One can assess this reality through observation. The observer is considered impartial and value free.	*Objectivist:* Same as for positivism, yet it is important to include perceptions of others, including those of the community.	*Transactional/ subjectivist:* Knowledge is mediated by values and specific contexts.	*Transactional/ subjectivist:* Knowledge is socially constructed by researchers and participants.	*Critical subjectivity:* It is important that experiences are shared, and that researchers and participants are part of a whole.
Methodology	*Experimental:* There is great reliance on observation. Factual knowledge can be gained by testing hypotheses.	*Modified experimental:* There is a need for multiple measures and observations (triangulation), as all observation is fallible.	*Dialogic/dialectical:* There is a reliance on dialogic methods (interviews, for example) that challenge assumptions.	*Hermeneutical/ dialectical:* Diverse methods are used to gain access to shared meanings as well as to expose conflicts, contradictions, and silences.	*Political participation:* A collaborative inquiry with a focus on action and self-awareness.

agencies, and communities add increasing pressures to further develop the field of community-based research.

In the face of these tensions, community members themselves are increasingly demanding that research reflect their needs and be applied to develop interventions; "the fundamental question is not about what knowledge is or is not but about what knowledge is for" (Trussler & Marchand, 2005, p. 45). While the evolution of community-based research reflects, at times, a considerable antagonism between practice and academia, it also has opened up the possibility that research can be more "understandable, responsive and pertinent to people's lives" (Flicker et al., 2008a, p. 107).

Although we are particularly interested in structuring this book to deal with community-based research, the debate and applicability of the arguments to work *with* communities are not limited to research. Indeed, the current tensions, challenges, and possibilities are also reflected in the fields of education and health care delivery. Community-based research provides a way to think about education, organizational learning, health care practices, and questions about institutional mandates and their relevance to community members, community organizations, and movements of resistance that seek self-determination. Questions about what ultimately improves the human condition are central to these debates. In the following chapter we turn to the principles of community-based research, where we differentiate community-based research from other research that is located within the community.

2. Community-based Research: Defining the Principles

I n the literature, there has been a tendency to conflate community-based research with participatory action research, community-based participatory research, and participatory research. In our work we have come to understand that community-based research represents a philosophical approach to the *conduct* of research, regardless of whether a qualitative or a quantitative methodology is used to answer the research question. Participatory action research, on the other hand, represents a specific methodology with a primary goal of prompting action, whether visible or invisible, as a result of the process or the findings. Although there are numerous similarities between community-based research, participatory research, and participatory action research, there are also a variety of differences.

Several authors (Cargo & Mercer, 2008; Macaulay et al., 2011) argue that "participatory research" is an umbrella term that includes community-based research, community-based participatory research, participatory action research, and other approaches to research that emphasize authentic community partnerships. In Table 2.1 we attempt to clarify the differences among these approaches. In this chapter we talk about the differences, make visible the way we situate community-based research, and then provide insights into the principles of community-based research using examples from our research.

As we reflect on these differences, we also know that the differences in approaches are at times difficult to recognize in the field. Judy Mill,

Essentials of Community-based Research by Vera Caine and Judy Mill, 23–34. © 2016 Left Coast Press, Inc. All rights reserved.

Table 2.1 Comparison of Approaches

	Viewpoint	Attention to Community Ethics	Capacity Building	Collaboration/ Authentic Engagement	Mutual Education	Taking Action	Knowledge Relevant to the Community
Community-based research	Approach	Yes	Yes	Yes	Yes	Not primary focus	Yes
Participatory research	Approach	Yes	Yes	Yes	Yes	Yes	Yes
Participatory action research	Methodology	Yes	Not primary focus	Yes	Not primary focus	Yes	Yes
Community-based participatory research	Approach or methodology	Yes	Yes	Yes	Yes	Yes	Yes
Traditional approach	Various methodologies	No	No	No	No	No	Not primary goal

with her colleagues Ameeta Singh, and Marliss Taylor (2012) used a community-based research approach to explore street-involved (such as women who were homeless), pregnant women's experiences in a prenatal program called "Women in the Shadows." Mill and Singh were invited by the community agency to inquire into the experiences using a qualitative approach. The "Women in the Shadows" program reported very positive outcomes using pregnancy support workers who shared a similar history with the clients. The workers had been pregnant and street-involved at some point in their lives. Stable housing was essential for the pregnant women; however, one of the greatest challenges was transitioning out of a street lifestyle. This work was grounded in a community-based approach and involved an evaluation of the program with a focus on the women's experiences of homelessness and accessing the program. The design and implementation of the research was negotiated with the community and involved both the women and the staff as research participants. This was important, as it made both the community agency and community members central to the research. The project was not designed to call forth action, although it was crucial to understand that the continuation of funding was under threat and that the research results could help to lobby for continuing funding.

Meredith Minkler and Nina Wallerstein (2008) argue that the various terminology used for participatory research can be traced to the geographical region where the research is carried out: the term "community-based participatory research" is frequently used in the United States; "community-based research" is the preferred term in Canada; and "action research" is more commonly used in the United Kingdom, Australia, and New Zealand. Most authors[1] argue that community-based participatory research is an approach or orientation to research; however, Strickland (2006) asserts that community-based participatory research could be either a philosophical approach or a method. Similarly, van de Sande and Schwartz (2011) argues that social work research should be carried out with a structural perspective to acknowledge the social, political, and economic factors that influence communities. These authors discussed both community-based research and participatory action research and suggested that community-based research brings with it a "different set of assumptions" (p. 59); however, these are not made explicit.

Principles of Community-based Research

Despite some differences between community-based research, participatory research, participatory action research, and community-based participatory research, they are all based on similar principles, including:

- Authentic engagement of researchers and community members (Garcia, Minkler, Cardenas, Grills, & Porter, 2014)
- Attention to the ethical implications of the research for individuals and communities (Kaufert et al., 2001)
- Adherence to collaboration (Jagosh et al., 2012)
- An attempt to balance the generalizable knowledge with benefits to the community (Jacquez, Vaughn, & Wagner, 2013)
- A focus on systems development (Wright, Roche, Von Unger, Block, & Gardner, 2010)
- A dedicated effort to integrate capacity building into the process by ensuring that the strengths and resources of team members and participants are valued (Mill et al., 2014b)
- Acknowledgment of the need for flexibility in the research design due to the iterative nature of the process

Reflecting on the "Women in the Shadows" research project, we can see the realization of principles of community-based research. Throughout the project the community agency staff remained central and the research assistant, who collected all of the research data, participated in the daily activities of the agency. The community agency had a history of integrating researchers in its operations who facilitated capacity building as well as the authentic engagement of researchers and community members. Yet, this approach also holds challenges and at times raises issues of loyalty. The community has a vested interest in demonstrating the benefits of the work, whereas the researchers might focus on generalizing knowledge or at other times be seen as too critical.

Research with Communities that Is Participatory

Community-based research is a cyclical and iterative research process that enables the integration of the researchers' methodological and theoretical expertise with the knowledge of non-academic partners (Cargo & Mercer, 2008). Community-based research is an approach to research that values authentic partnerships with community members. The generation of knowledge relevant to the community and attention to building the capacity of community partners are fundamental tenets of this approach.

Participatory research is based on principles that are very closely aligned with community-based research. Mutual respect and trust are the core elements of participatory research and are necessary to support the goals of capacity building, empowerment, and ownership (Cargo & Mercer, 2008). Jagosh and colleagues (2012) define participatory research as an approach that encompasses "the co-construction of research between researchers and the people affected by the issues under study" (p. 312). These authors conducted a systematic appraisal to assess the outcomes of 23 participatory partnerships and reported that partnership synergy tended to result in research that was culturally appropriate and logistically realistic; generated recruitment capacity; developed the capacity and competence of stakeholders; created increasingly positive outcomes; enhanced sustainability; and generated systemic changes. Macaulay and colleagues (1999) conducted an integrated review of the literature and suggest that in addition to collaboration and mutual education, taking action and promoting social change are also goals of participatory research.

Participatory action research as a methodology shares many similarities with a community-based research approach. Loewenson and colleagues (2014) recently published a reader that traces the history of participatory action research, examining key features of this approach and exploring its use to improve health systems. These authors suggest that researchers using a participatory action research methodology attempt to challenge power imbalances to act on social determinants, change health systems, and achieve greater social justice. To do this, researchers typically bring together partners that include representatives from communities, researchers, and policy and decision makers. The authors argue that one characteristic that differentiates participatory action research from other participatory approaches is that participatory action research is "deeply linked to socio-political processes, such as the popular education movement in Latin America, Asia, and Africa" (Loewenson et al., 2014, p. 16).

In the "Women in the Shadows" project, the link to sociopolitical processes was not made explicit. It was difficult to trace the project to issues of social justice, and the researchers did not intentionally attempt to challenge power imbalances. Yet, the project was a vehicle to challenge possible funding cuts and shift public opinion about pregnant women who use substances. As a result of this project we realized that each research project must be understood within the context of participating researchers or community agencies. In this instance Judy Mill, Ameeta Singh, and the agency had a long history of addressing the social determinants of health and working with vulnerable and marginalized populations. We have come to know how important it is to understand not only the process of collaboration, but also to establish a shared philosophy. At the same time, it is critical to know who the community is.

Returning to Defining Community

As we point out earlier, despite the acknowledged benefits of including community members in the research, there may be disagreements about how the community is defined and who represents the community (Israel, Schulz, Parker, & Becker, 1998). DeSantis (2014) reminds us that community-based research is not a neutral approach, "but a value-laden exercise based on a model of research *with* communities not research *about* communities" (p. 55; italics added). Denise Drevdahl (2002) also explores the concept of community and argues that the process of defining membership in a community is complex and is dependent on the context. She cautions against "subsuming differences under a framework of unity" (p. 10) to form community. The process of suppressing differences in identity results in the formation of borders and the development of border communities (Drevdahl, 2002).

We agree with the premise that community can include any individual or organization that shares with the researcher an interest in the topic under study or is affected by the issue (Macaulay & Nutting, 2006). To ensure the breadth and depth of knowledge required, academic researchers involved in community-based research should represent a range of disciplines and expertise (Cargo & Mercer, 2008). The non-academic community partners can refer to a wide range of individuals who work alongside the academic researcher(s) and can include community members and leaders, patients and clients, the support network of clients, community-based health professionals, policy- and decision-makers, and representatives from community-based organizations. Margaret Cargo and Shawna Mercer (2008) have developed a list of questions to help the research team identify who should be invited to participate in the community-based research partnership.

Depending on the leadership within communities, universities and funders paradoxically may have more control over who represents the community than do community organizations (Wallerstein & Duran, 2006). For example, a funder or university-based ethics review board may negatively assess a research project if they do not understand the rationale for the inclusion of various community partners. Israel and colleagues (2008) remind us that academics must be careful not to define who represents the community, while at the same time considering who has the time and skills to participate in the research and who has influence in the community. Plumb, Price, and Kavanaugh-Lynch (2004) reviewed several community-based research projects to encourage breast cancer research with hard-to-research Californian women. Although they identify many benefits to this approach, they report that the greatest weakness was engaging the broad community outside of the research team.

Community-placed or Community-based

Meredith Minkler and Nina Wallerstein (2008) highlight the increasing demand for community-based participatory research and advocate for research that is "community-based rather than merely community-placed" (p. 5). Similarly, Macaulay and Nutting (2006) argue that community-based research is different from other research in which the community is viewed only as a place or location. Jacquez and colleagues (2013) conducted a review of community-based participatory research related to youth and found that despite many authors stating they had used this approach, many studies were community placed rather than community based and partnered with adults rather than children. The authors emphasize that community-based participatory research must have not only have a participatory component but also align with the principles of collaboration and engagement.

Establishing Partnerships

Establishing authentic partnerships between academic and community members who are part of the research team is fundamental to community-based research. These partnerships require time and patience (Stoecker, 2008); however, there has been limited research to evaluate the effect of participation on health outcomes (Wallerstein & Duran, 2006). Margaret Cargo and Shawna Mercer (2008) suggest that there are four stages to the establishment of partnerships: engagement, formalization, mobilization, and maintenance. The roles and responsibilities of the research team members differ depending on the stage of partnerships. The level of participation in participatory research is dynamic, occurs along a continuum, and must be continuously negotiated; when academic researchers share power with community members, "empowering co-investigation" (Chung & Lounsbury, 2006, p. 2132) is possible. We have also found that the level of participation of both community and academic partners varies depending on the phase of the research. This is consistent with the findings of other researchers (Minkler, 2004; Ross et al., 2010) who have asserted that participation and involvement may vary depending on the expertise and time available for each partner. In the project "Women in the Shadows," the involvement of the community agency was much greater at the beginning of the project and during the data collection. The researchers were the primary data analysts; the community agency played a more consultative role.

Ann Macaulay and Paul Nutting (2006) extend the notion of partnerships by advocating for partnerships between researchers, clinicians, and the recipients of the clinical practice. The recipients of the clinical practice could include both patients and family members. Some academics believe that engaging with community members may be a double-edged sword. For example, involving community members in the research process may lead to biased research (Nyden, 2003). Despite this concern, it has become standard practice in our research to include people living with HIV on both research teams and community advisory committees. In fact, in many countries it would be difficult to receive funding without one or more people living with HIV as part of the team. This is a recognition of the principles that call for the greater involvement of people living with AIDS (GIPA; Joint United Nations Programme on HIV/AIDS [UNAIDS], 1999).

Partnerships within community-based research are mutually beneficial and reflect "a profound belief in partnership synergy" (Minkler, 2005, p. ii4). Partnership synergy refers to the phenomenon in which organizations can achieve more by working together than they can by working alone (Lasker, Weiss, & Miller, 2001). Lasker and colleagues argue that there has been limited description of the process through which partnerships influence outcomes; however, they suggest that synergy is "the proximal outcome of partnership functioning that gives collaboration a unique advantage" (p. 183) over single agents. These authors argue that collaboration can generate creative, comprehensive, practical, and transformative thinking and propose a framework to assess the effectiveness of partnership synergy.

We have found that experienced community partners are able to provide wise counsel in relation to the ebb and flow of the research process, including the involvement of team members. A unique challenge in the conduct of community-based research is that community organizational partners may face a burden to participate in research without adequate time and resources while continuing to provide services.[2] Therefore, it is important to consider interests, expertise, and available time when determining the participation level of the academic and non-academic partners (Cargo & Mercer, 2008). Plumb and colleagues (2004) report that some community partners also experience an increased demand for their services as a result of their participation in research.

Regardless of the name, community-based research demands a consultative approach with individuals and communities; in some research projects the community will choose to actively participate in all or some aspects of the research, whereas in others they may prefer to continue in a consultative role throughout the process. As the name implies, individuals and communities actively participate when a participatory action research methodology is used. Research that combines both a community-based approach and participatory methodology implies both consultation and participation (Mill et al., 2014b; Strickland, 2006).

Is Community-based Research Appropriate for All Types of Research?

As we mentioned, community-based research can be used as an approach for all types of research. Community-based research is appropriate for research with diverse populations and is particularly congruent for research with Indigenous communities. We argue that community-based research is an essential approach for research with Indigenous[3] communities because it is congruent with the principles of ownership, control, access, and possession (OCAP™; Schnarch, 2004) that are foundational to Indigenous research. In addition, participatory community-based research is a culturally appropriate approach (Strickland, 2006) that has the potential to honor both Indigenous and academic communities by adhering to the principles of decolonizing methodologies (Stanton, 2014). (See chapter 8 of this book for additional discussion on research with Indigenous communities.)

Community-based research is also an appropriate approach with a wide range of communities and populations. In Toronto a community-based research approach was used to explore the sexual and ethnic identities of Black gay men, including the challenges they faced in participating in HIV research (George et al., 2012). Flicker (2008) led a community-based research project to train HIV-positive youth and service providers in the design, implementation, and data analysis of needs with HIV-positive Ontario youth. In a review of youth involvement in community-based participatory research, Jacquez and colleagues (2013) remind us that although it is less common for youth to be research partners, their unique voice is essential to ensure that their context is understood and considered throughout the research process. Charlotte Chang and her colleagues (2013) used a community-based approach to explore factors, structures, and processes that facilitated the integration and participation of Chinese immigrant workers in San Francisco.

Community-based research is also particularly relevant and useful to research with populations who live with inequities[4] or are culturally diverse (Strickland, 2006). Sarah Flicker (2008), who is well known in Canada for her in community-based research and community development, reported that HIV-positive youth involvement in a community-based project provided an opportunity for them to be actively engaged in a respected activity, which in turn enhanced their self-esteem. Nearly all of the youth in Flicker's study were current or previous members of one or more communities that were socially excluded (e.g., homeless, intravenous drug users, or gay). Garcia and colleagues (2014) also report that with consistent adult mentors, youth who lack stability have the necessary skills to contribute to policy-focused community-based participatory research.

Challenges and Opportunities

The benefits of using a community-based research approach are both tangible and intangible. To realize the benefits, there must be a considerable investment of human and financial resources (Flicker, 2008) and an understanding of the challenges inherent to community-based research:

- **Increased time** to carry out ethically sound community-based research (Flicker, 2008; Flicker et al., 2008b; Israel et al., 1998; Katz & Martin, 1997; Macaulay et al., 1999; Martz & Bacsu, 2014; Stanton, 2014; Strickland, 2006).

- **Additional project costs** related to the increased time required to administer the research projects, negotiate different research cultures, understand new value systems, and learn a variety of financial systems (Katz & Martin, 1997). In Flicker's community-based research project with HIV-positive youth (2008), participants believed that although the emphasis on process and collaboration contributed to its success, these elements also resulted in the project taking longer. Flicker also identified role confusion and loss of control as additional costs related to engagement.
- **Obtaining funding and achieving tenure and promotion,** both related to the time commitment, have been cited as major challenges by academics who are engaged with community-based research (Israel et al., 1998; Jones & Wells, 2007; MacLean, Warr, & Pyett, 2009; Wallerstein & Duran, 2006). To help faculty overcome this challenge, Seifer (2008) describes the characteristics of quality community-engaged scholarship and develops guidelines for individuals to prepare for their institution's review of their work.
- **Power differentials** are another challenge to community-based research (Chung & Lounsbury, 2006; Flicker, 2008; Flicker, Travers, Guta, McDonald, & Meagher, 2007; Israel et al., 1998; London, 2007; Marshall, Peterson, Coverdale, Etzel, & McFarland, 2014; van de Sande & Schwartz, 2011). DeSantis (2014) reminds us that power can operate both negatively to create imbalances and positively to promote advocacy for change. Power differentials among members of the research team, community partners, and individuals responsible for knowledge dissemination may be problematic and result in poorer outcomes.
- **Differential reward structures** among team members with academic researchers gaining more from the collaboration (Minkler, 2004, 2005). Chung and Lounsbury (2006) argue that "failing to resolve divergent assumptions about power and purpose can lead to fissures that are difficult to overcome" (p. 2129). Similarly, Flicker (2008) reminds us that despite the benefits of community-based research, "those benefits might accrue differentially across power structures and are not without substantial costs" (p. 71). She argues that the benefits and challenges of community-based research must be examined critically on an ongoing basis.

Despite the challenge related to increased time, community-based research has the potential to encourage community development and promote mutually respectful partnerships between academic and community members. In addition to building the confidence of individuals, the empowerment of organizations and communities is possible through a community-based research approach (Minkler, 2005). Another advantage of community-based research is that this approach may help to break down the disciplinary turf boundaries that are common in universities (Nyden, 2003) and to influence and change policy (Themba-Nixon, Minkler, & Freudenberg, 2008). Solina Richter and colleagues (2013) recently reported findings from a project that explored the influence of workplace policies on nursing care for individuals and families living with HIV in Jamaica, Kenya, South Africa, and Uganda. Although nurses in all of the participating countries commented on their lack of involvement in policy development, their participation in the community-based research process highlighted the urgent need for them to become involved in the formulation of HIV policy.

Community-based research also has the potential to contribute to higher-quality research, including the design of interventions that are congruent with the values and needs of the community (Flicker, 2008; Nyden, 2003). Nyden (2003) suggests that community-based research may actually provide political value for universities because they are able to demonstrate to their funders that their research is relevant and beneficial to local communities. Flicker (2008) evaluated the benefits of a community-based research project with HIV-positive youth and reported that the approach led to better questions, recruitment, data collection, analysis, dissemination, and action and resulted in benefits to the stakeholders, including HIV-positive youth, academics, and service providers.

Community-based research represents an attempt to overcome some of the tensions that occur in traditional approaches to research, including some communities' lack of trust in research, the tendency to undervalue community knowledge, the lack of community inclusion in the dissemination of findings, and limited opportunities for communities to generate knowledge (Plumb, Price, & Kavanaugh-Lynch, 2004). As we think once more about "Women in the Shadows," we can see how important it was to design the project as a community-based research project. Using this approach, the research team was able to work alongside peer support workers from the community partner organization to engage women who were extremely vulnerable, homeless, and pregnant to become active participants in their prenatal care.

In the next chapter, we provide an in-depth exploration of two community-based research projects to demonstrate the link between their philosophical and theoretical foundations and the practice of implementing community-based research.

Section II
The Practice of Community-based Research

3. From Theory to Practice

Over the years we have participated in a number of different community-based research projects. In this chapter we highlight two different projects. We chose these projects to demonstrate the connection between the theoretical underpinnings and the practices of community-based research. In particular we focus on the research processes, rather than the outcomes or findings of each project. Each research project differs in terms of the origin of the research question(s), the purpose of the research, the involvement of the community of interest, the scope of the project, and the handling of disagreements. We will highlight some of these differences, not as a way to delineate one right or best way to undertake projects, but to show that each project also has a life of its own that is often unpredictable. We chose the "Challenging Lifestyles: Aboriginal Men and Women Living with HIV" (Mill, Lambert, Larkin,

Essentials of Community-based Research by Vera Caine and Judy Mill, 35–47. © 2016 Left Coast Press, Inc. All rights reserved.

Ward, & Harrowing, 2007) and the Délı̨nę Uranium Research (Canada-Délı̨nę Uranium Table [CDUT], 2005) projects for this purpose.

Challenging Lifestyles

The research study "Challenging Lifestyles: Aboriginal Men and Women Living with HIV" was carried out between September 2002 and November 2004 with funding from Health Canada through the Aboriginal Community-Based Research Program of the Canadian Strategy on HIV/AIDS. The goal of research was first to explore the experiences of Aboriginal persons living with HIV in the period following diagnosis to identify factors that limited or enhanced risky behavior, and in a second phase to design an intervention to promote healthier lifestyles for Aboriginal persons living with HIV. These goals were consistent with two of the goals of the Canadian Strategy on HIV/AIDS to prevent the spread of HIV infection in Canada and to ensure care, treatment, and support for Canadians living with AIDS.

Origin of the Research Question

The research question reflected part of Judy Mill's larger program of research. She was interested in HIV-related stigma (Mill et al., 2009) both in the Aboriginal population and for women in international settings, such as Ghana (Mill, 2003; Mill & Anarfi, 2002). Judy was immersed in the academic literature as well as in ongoing conversations with community members. As a result of this experience, the research question crystallized. At the time of the research, HIV prevention strategies focused primarily on the interruption of the disease before infection. At the same time, there was an increased recognition of the need to investigate factors that increased or limited the spread of the virus in infected individuals (Schiltz & Sandfort, 2000). Several excellent harm reduction programs, such as needle exchanges and condom distribution, existed in Alberta (a western province in Canada) to prevent the spread of HIV and other infectious diseases. Despite these programs, community members of the research team were concerned that HIV-seropositive individuals did not always use them. Anecdotal information suggested that access was a major barrier to the participation of Aboriginal individuals in harm reduction programs; however, limited research had been done in Alberta to explore this problem.

Purpose of the Research

After many conversations with members of the research team, it became clear that in the first phase of the study we needed to examine the experiences of HIV-positive Aboriginal individuals in Alberta in the period following diagnosis to identify factors that limited or enhanced risky behavior. Within a community-based research approach, the research team chose participatory action research as the design for the study, using in-depth interviews as the primary data collection method. During the second phase of the study, the team planned an intervention to promote healthier lifestyles for Aboriginal persons living with HIV. However, because of the length of time it took to complete the first phase of the study, and the recognition that HIV stigma was still extremely high in Aboriginal communities in rural Alberta, we revisited the initial intervention plan. In consultation with the Community Advisory Committee (discussed shortly), the research team developed and led a skills-building workshop for individuals living with HIV, some of whom had been research participants. In addition, the team presented the findings from the first phase in several rural communities in Alberta. The communities were extremely interested in the findings related to the challenging lifestyles participants experienced, and the research team felt these presentations were interventions in themselves. The ability to be flexible in the research design and implementation is one of the principles of community-based research.

Involvement of the Community of Interest

This project brought together research team members and organizations with the varied and relevant backgrounds required to complete the research. Members of Kimamow Atoskanow Foundation, a community-based organization committed to the provision of HIV prevention programs and support services to Aboriginal individuals, families, and communities throughout Alberta, worked with faculty at the University of Alberta to provide guidance for the overall management of the project. Denise Lambert, the executive director of the Kimamow Atoskanow Foundation, and Kecia Larkin and Ken Ward, longstanding members of Kimamow, were co-investigators on the research project from the development of the proposal to the dissemination of the findings. Their grassroots experience in HIV prevention and support initiatives for individuals and communities across Canada, in combination with their life experiences as Aboriginal people, ensured that the research project was culturally sound.

In addition to the members of the research team, a Community Advisory Committee provided advice and guidance throughout the project. The Community Advisory Committee members were selected by the community research partners based on their knowledge of HIV in Aboriginal communities, and included an elder and two Aboriginal persons living with HIV. The research team, including the research assistant and the Community Advisory Committee members, used their extensive relationships and networks with individuals, families, communities, and organizations to inform and recruit individuals to the study. These networks were critical to the success of the project.

Judy assumed the overall responsibility for ensuring that the terms of the Contribution Agreement between Health Canada and the research team were met and the financial reporting requirements completed. She also ensured that the project received ethical approval, not only from the University of Alberta Health Research Ethics Board, but also from the Community Advisory Committee. The ethics review by the Community Advisory Committee focused on the impact of the project from a community perspective, and involved evaluating the project to ensure it was culturally sound and respectful toward the individuals and communities involved.

Dr. Stan Houston, the second academic member of the team, brought valuable and unique expertise to the team. He is a senior physician in General Internal Medicine and Infectious Diseases at the University of Alberta Hospital, Edmonton, and holds an academic appointment as a professor. Dr. Houston is recognized for his contributions to the care and treatment of individuals with HIV in northern Alberta, particularly in diverse populations. He assisted the research team to identify individuals, agencies, and communities that were interested in participating in the research and provided ongoing input as a member of the research team.

Once ethical approval was obtained, Judy and two community research team members recruited a research coordinator and research assistant to assist with project management and oversee data collection and analysis during the project. The research assistant (James Makokis) was a student at the University of Alberta and was himself Aboriginal. All the interviews that James completed were in depth, respectful, and reflected his deep knowledge of Aboriginal communities. Throughout the project all members of the research team were involved in the data collection as well as the analysis process. Based on the extremely powerful initial findings related to the stigma and discrimination experienced by participants, the Community Advisory Committee recommended sharing these findings with communities in northern Alberta. Because many of these communities were reluctant to discuss HIV and AIDS publicly owing to stigma, these presentations were themselves a meaningful intervention.

Presentations on the research study were carried out with health workers, community members, and community leaders in several Alberta communities. The purpose of the presentations was not only to present the research findings, but also to share the research process. The involvement of Aboriginal people living with HIV was an integral part of the intervention, and therefore Kimamow organized a workshop to provide presentation skills training to Aboriginal people living with HIV. Individuals living with HIV from three of the communities in Alberta who assisted with the recruitment of participants were invited to attend the training session. Some of those who attended the workshops were also participants in the study. One of these participants, Douglas Gauld, participated in many of the community presentations with the research team to ensure that the voices of Aboriginal people living with HIV were heard. Douglas's involvement in the project became a turning point in his life. He spoke to the team about his desire to give back to Aboriginal communities, and after his participation in the project he wrote a book about his life experiences and became involved with Aboriginal HIV community support organizations.

Scope of the Project

The scope of the project broadened when members of the research team realized that the dissemination of the findings was in itself the intervention. Several recommendations were made from the study based on the participants' comments, the analysis of the data, and the guidance of the Community Advisory Committee. To improve the experience of Aboriginal persons living with HIV the team recommended: (1) providing support; (2) acknowledging the challenging lifestyles of individuals; (3) decreasing stigma and discrimination; (4) ensuring equitable access to services; (5) integrating traditional healers and elders; and (6) promoting a holistic approach to health. To improve HIV prevention and care in Aboriginal communities, the team also recommended: (1) increasing education; (2) supporting positive role models; and (3) providing additional resources.

While the findings continued to be shared through the ongoing community work of Kimamow Atoskanow Foundation, the findings also informed new research projects. This was facilitated by our commitment to continuing relationships following the completion of the project and recognition that each team member brought unique skills and expertise to the research topic. Both of us (Judy Mill and Vera Caine) have continued to work alongside Ken Ward in research projects subsequent to "Challenging Lifestyles." For example, we have invited Ken to share his deep understanding about HIV in Aboriginal communities with nurses who wish to increase their knowledge about HIV. At the same time, we acknowledged the importance of using more traditional formats for dissemination, such as presentations at national and international conferences and articles in journals as important strategies to influence policy.

Handling Disagreements

Disagreements in this project were handled by reaching consensus among all members of the research team, as well as in consultation with the Community Advisory Committee. Over the course of the project, however, Judy learned that Aboriginal team members preferred to handle tensions and disagreements in a less direct manner, preferably using a face-to-face approach. Therefore, when Judy felt that a discussion was likely to be controversial, she would discuss it with Denise Lambert in person before a research team or Community Advisory Committee meeting to get advice on how best to deal with the issue. Important in this process was that all people were clear about the overall goal of the project. As Channing Crowshoe, one of the Community Advisory Committee members, said:

> I would like to say how much I have learned sitting on the Advisory Committee in regards to OCAP™ [Ownership, Control, Access, and Possession] of information. This project has proved to me that a group as diverse as ours *can* work together for the betterment of all people. Oftentimes we are divided by cultural and territorial boundaries that have the potential to conquer and defeat us all. I must say that it has been a pleasure to be a part of this project and I will continue to carry it in my heart, mind and prayers. (Channing Crowshoe, personal communication, March 2004)

James Makokis, the research assistant for the project, also made it evident that the often-artificial boundaries between friend and colleague can become blurred. This blurring was significant in this project, in which many of the friendships between academic and community partners still continue today. This blurriness is essential to the process of community-based research. As James pointed out:

"Challenging Lifestyles" has been a wonderful project to be involved with and I am very fortunate to have been selected as the research assistant over the course of its duration. When I was hired, I was an undergraduate student and viewed research and the research process as being somewhat limited. My perception was confined to the conventional image of a scientist working in a white lab coat, in a lab, studying rats. After being introduced to the project, my perception of research changed dramatically. Instead of working with rats, I was able to talk with people and had the honor of listening to their stories about their life and about living with HIV. I learned much from talking with the study participants: about their lives, challenges, struggles, lessons, and also about the more positive influences that occurred as a result of their diagnosis. I also learned a lot about myself: about the importance of valuing life, living each day to the fullest, nurturing existing relationships, while fostering the development of new ones. I am humbled and most thankful for being given the opportunity to have a glimpse into such magnificent peoples' lives. This research project brought together a group of people with whom I am glad to now call friends and colleagues. Watching the compassion and commitment that others have for improving the collective good of Aboriginal people was motivating and refreshing, for it is through collaboration and cooperation that we can accomplish much more than if we work individually. *Ay ay* [thank you]. (James Makokis, personal communication, March 2004)

The research team and the Community Advisory Committee members felt that the project was very effective in unveiling the very challenging lifestyles that the research participants had experienced before and after their HIV diagnoses. In addition, after the project James Makokis continued his education and is now a physician, Denise Lambert pursued graduate education, and Douglas Gould wrote a book about his life. Although these positive stories and participation in the project cannot be directly linked, it is likely that the research project had some unintended positive outcomes.

41

Délınę Uranium Research

The Délınę Uranium Research project was very different in its process than the "Challenging Lifestyles" project. The Délınę Uranium Research project is situated within a long and ongoing history of the community of Délınę (previously called Fort Franklin) in the Northwest Territories in Canada. Vera Caine became part of this research when she and her family moved to the community, where her partner had been invited to conduct his doctoral research. Vera still recalls her first time in the small fly-in community in a remote part of northern Canada; the community was located just below the treeline on the shores of one of the largest freshwater lakes in the world. The community was seeking someone for a position on a research project who had a background in the health sciences and was also familiar with communities in the Northwest Territories. Before accepting the position and congruent with the principles of community-based research, Vera engaged in conversations with community members to see if this was a good fit for everyone. Vera was involved in the project from 2003 to 2004 as the Health and Social Research Coordinator. The primary goal of the research was to address the impact of a radium and uranium mine that operated from 1931 to 1960 on the eastern shores of Great Bear Lake through discrete research studies that explored the environmental as well as health and social impacts. Many Dene men had been employed as ore carriers at the mine, or were family members who lived close to the transportation route. Dene people did not learn about the environmental and health effects of radium and uranium exposure until the 1980s. In 1998, the following news release was issued:

We, the Sahtugot'ine (the Dene of Great Bear Lake) have been subjected to and continue to suffer from a grave injustice imposed on us by the Canadian government. Without being told of the deadly hazards of radiation, our men carried radioactive ore and our families and children have been exposed to radiation for over 60 years. We are concerned, in particular, about:

1) The deaths of our community members from cancer and other radiation and mining related diseases and the psychological and social impact these deaths of have had on us; and,
2) the presence of millions of tons of radioactive waste in our Great Bear Lake environment, which we regard as our source of food and spiritual nourishment. (Canadian Coalition for Nuclear Responsibility, 1998)

The statement, released well before the release of the final report from the research that was ultimately undertaken, provides a glimpse into the long history of the issue. Yet the statement remains relevant today and highlights the grave injustices uranium mining on Great Bear Lake has brought to the community of Délı̨nę: past, present, and future. While the community continues to feel the immediate impact, it is important to also acknowledge the larger social implications of uranium mining at Great Bear Lake. The uranium harvested from what became known as the Port Radium mine was used in the bombing of Hiroshima; community members have always felt a sense of responsibility for these events and have traveled to Japan to apologize for their involvement in mining or transportation activities. These transportation activities are also referred to as "the highway of the atom" (van Wyck, 2010).

Origin of the Research Question

In the 1980s, community members in Délı̨nę learned about the impact of radium and uranium mining; up until that time, the Canadian Government had been largely silent about this impact. During this time, the community also experienced significant losses of their older men, many who were regarded as elders within the community. In 1998, Peter Blow produced a one-hour documentary titled *Village of Widows*, which

> chronicles the Sahtu Dene peoples' struggle to come to terms with the mine's legacy, and its lasting impact on their traditional homeland on the shores of Canada's Great Bear Lake. It concludes with a remarkable display of humanity, when a group from Délı̨nę traveled to Hiroshima to meet Japanese bomb survivors. (Blow, 1998)

This documentary, together with increasing pressure from within the community of Délı̨nę forced the federal government to investigate the concerns raised. Unlike other academic research approaches, in this community-based research project the community identified the research questions, secured funding, and also was invested heavily in the outcome of the research.

Purpose of the Research

In 1999, the Canada-Délı̨nę Uranium Table (CDUT) was formed between the federal government and the Délı̨nę First Nation to address the environmental and human health impacts caused by the radium and uranium mine. In the following year, meetings involving community members and experts were held to determine a three-year action plan that delineated research studies and activities that "would provide the information necessary to enable the community of Délı̨nę and the federal government to make informed decisions about the Port Radium mine site and any community health issues relating to the mine" (CDUT, 2005, p. ii).

Involvement of the Community of Interest

Reflecting upon the history of Délı̨nę it is evident that without the commitment of community members to act upon the community's concerns, the research projects undertaken to determine a three-year plan would have never occurred. The community formed the Délı̨nę Uranium Committee in 1998 (Délı̨nę First Nations, 2005a), which began to collect oral histories almost immediately. For the community, the collection of oral histories was critical as they faced the loss of several community members. As Danny Gaudet (cited in Markey, 2005) pointed out, "It was a community process to provide answers that have been unanswered for too long." Over the course of several years community members were trained not only in ways to conduct the oral histories, but also how to transcribe the interviews in North Slavey (the language spoken in the Aboriginal community),[1] translate these into English, and engage in analysis processes. The long-term benefits of engaging in a community-based research project for the community was the systematic development of the capacity to speak and write in North Slavey and to provide translation between North Slavey and English.

When the official plan and research initiatives were formed, one of the goals was also to build capacity within the community. It was critical not only to build capacity in undertaking and leading research projects but also to ensure that the overall project sustained its necessary community leadership. Throughout the project, 32 community members were directly employed, while many others provided support or were hired through contract work in numerous roles. In this community-based research project the roles of community members included, for example, interviewers, translators, and research assistants collecting and processing biological samples of caribou and fish, among others; community members also provided the oversight, leadership, and administration, as well as led communication efforts.

As the various research projects unfolded, it was important that researchers were able to communicate in North Slavey. This was particularly relevant in the cornerstone project on traditional knowledge, for which it was necessary to establish a comprehensive database of traditional activities, hunting routes, and maps as well as the activities undertaken by ore carriers and their families since the 1930s. The ability to speak North Slavey and to understand cultural protocols embedded in language also became evident as researchers and community members interacted in research activities, public presentations, and discussions about the significance of the research findings. While the ability to speak multiple languages is not necessary for all community-based research projects, it was essential for this project. Elders in the community, who only spoke North Slavey, guided researchers in knowledge of cultural protocols and acceptable ways to engage in research. Research activities also needed to be explained to researchers who were not from the community and did not speak North Slavey. To widen the impact of the research, all final research results were communicated in North Slavey and English. As part of this community training, a program for community fieldworkers was established and involved formalized educational programs with academic credits. Community members were also involved in environmental monitoring research as field guides and through work experiences in schools.

The leadership for the project involved key community members, including the chief land claims negotiator for the community, as well as the manager and communications manager. A close connection existed throughout the project between the chief negotiator, staff, the Délı̨nę First Nations Chief and Council, and advisors. Because all of the research offices and activities were coordinated through the community, researchers were easily accessible to community members and were regular participants in the daily life of the community.

Scope of the Project

The scope of the overall work of the CDUT was extensive; it was important for everyone to understand how each individual research project connected to the overall work and goals of the community. Several of the individual research projects were led by researchers from outside of the community who did not always understand how projects related to each other and therefore missed important opportunities to further the overall goal. One of the more successful examples is when the oral history project was turned into a book that was printed and distributed within the community and to some extent across Canada. In this case community members identified that moving forward in good ways was important to them; moving forward included ensuring that many people learned about the history of Délı̨nę. Within each research project, the community—and particularly the leadership of the CDUT—made sure that community members participated to their full capacity and that researchers offered activities to build and sustain capacities.

While the goal of the project was to develop a three-year action plan and to answer the questions the community had in relation to the impact of radium and uranium mining, it was also important that the project stemmed from the community's social and political agenda. As Merine MacKeinzo (as cited in Délı̨nę First Nations, 2005a) points out:

> We can't just leave our land. We want a bright future for our children and we want to raise them well. We use the whole land for hunting. It is pitiful how they spoiled that part of the land. The Dene people worked in a dangerous setting without knowing, but they still worked. While they worked the wind must have blown the ore dust in the air and the people breathed it in and they also drank polluted water. So when I think about everything that happened I don't like it. At that time our people didn't speak English. The White people probably knew about the dangers involved but didn't say anything.

Handling Disagreements

Throughout the overall project, individual research projects were developed and many of the projects were implemented in different ways depending on their intention and scope. As requests for proposals were developed for these projects, the CDUT operated on an understanding of consensus and mutual respect. Community members and representatives from the federal government reviewed proposals for the projects before the work could proceed. While this was a process that appeared to reflect diverse interests, it also became clear that not all researchers who undertook research or assisted with capacity building within the community were familiar with the cultural and community protocols. The community eventually developed ethical guidelines for research and also outlined more specific guidelines relevant to natural resource management in a document titled *Dene Ways of Respecting the Land and Animals* (Délı̨nę First Nations, 2005b). The principles outlined in these guidelines aimed at finding balance between the present and future and respecting the interrelationship between the land, animals, and people. The guidelines and protocols were developed with community members, written in North Slavey and English, and became ways in which to navigate disagreements.

Over the course of the project, community members, researchers, and government representatives developed mutual understandings of assessing the results of the overall project. While individual scientific projects were guided by different methodologies and assessed based on the rigor and validity of individual methods, the overall project was assessed differently. The community and government representatives engaged in joint meetings to develop recommendations to address the findings.

Reflections

Both studies were located in Canada, which has a long history in community-based research. The studies demonstrate the link between community members, community agencies or political bodies, and advocacy as strategies to address identified concerns. The two studies also provide an opportunity to compare approaches to community-based research. While both projects were complex, the project in the community of Délı̨nę consisted of several research studies with various methodological approaches to achieve the goals of the community. From the beginning it was clear that the project in Délı̨nę had a strong political and social justice agenda, and was very much focused on democratizing knowledge. The "Challenging Lifestyles" project was a single study that reflected an agreed-upon academic and community goal. The scope of the analysis and the link to practices within communities involved community members who were both co-investigators and members of the advisory board. Both projects required a significant amount of collaboration and a willingness to work through disagreements; relationship and capacity building were essential. The impact of each project was significantly greater because of the community-based approach. One of the significant elements of community-based research is the need to pay close attention to the overall research design, which is the focus of the next chapter.

4. Research Design

As we look across our projects, we are aware of how our understanding of community-based research has changed over time. Some of our understanding has been shaped by others we engage with in community-based research, but also by being part of discussions with academic and community members while making decisions about funding, as we teach methodology and research courses in our university, and through seminars or workshops with community members. We have made several observations during the implementation of our community-based research projects: *methodological plurality* is a key design element when using this approach; methodological decisions in community-based research *reflect political and social influences*; and *rigor* in community-based research needs to be better developed and understood to reflect the inherently rich contributions community-based research can make without compromising scientific merit.

Methodological Plurality

The Délįnę Uranium Research project is a particularly good example of research that calls for methodological plurality to answer several distinct research questions. As part of the project, several studies were proposed and conducted, including an oral history project that involved ethnographic work to document people's involvement as ore carriers; an epidemiological study that involved calculating detailed historical exposure to radiation for ore transport workers and their families; and environmental sampling studies, site assessments, and ecological risk assessments. Each study called forth a diverse range of study designs and different methodologies

Essentials of Community-based Research by Vera Caine and Judy Mill, 49–59. © 2016 Left Coast Press, Inc. All rights reserved.

with sometimes the same and sometimes different methods. As Meredith Minkler (2005), one of the key U.S.-based community-based researchers, points out, "[community-based participatory research] is not a method per se but an orientation to research that may employ any of a number of qualitative and quantitative methodologies" (p. ii). In the Délı̨nę Uranium Research project, each discrete study informed other studies and at the same time was always connected to the larger goal of the project.

While it is critical to understand that community-based research can employ both qualitative and quantitative approaches, it is important to recognize that the epistemological and ontological foundations of community-based research are still inseparable from methodological decisions. This is an important point, particularly if community members are involved in all stages of the research, including selecting the study design, securing funding, implementing the study, analyzing and interpreting the data, disseminating findings, translating research into practice and policy, and sustaining the team, benefits, and resources (Horowitz, Robinson, & Seifer, 2009). It is our experience that community members who are involved in community-based research rarely lose sight of the overall goal or its potential impact; however, it is challenging to be equally involved in all of stages of a community-based research project. Sarah Flicker and colleagues (2008b) report that "community members were most often involved in defining research questions, collecting data and using the findings for advocacy purposes. They were least likely to be involved in data analysis and interpretation" (p. 112). To be closely involved in the study selection and design stage, community members who may be unfamiliar with all research methodologies need the opportunity to develop their capacity. Vera recalls that it was critical for community members to understand oral history methodologies as well as the methods involved in reconstructing the historical exposure to radiation. Without understanding these approaches it was difficult for community members to identify potential participants or to develop questions they felt were relevant to ask, or engage in more critical aspects of the data analysis and dissemination.

It is equally important to build capacity for researchers situated in academia. Making methodological choices without knowing about the people, cultures, and settings of a research project can be detrimental, particularly as assumptions about transferability are made (Cargo & Mercer, 2008). Decisions about methodologies and subsequently about methods must reflect the considerations made about barriers to participation (such as linguistic difference, which was present in the Délı̨nę Uranium Research project) within communities and about how data will be accessible to the community and academic team members during and after the completion of a research project. Issues of confidentiality alongside power and control may be at stake in projects when, for example, participants who may be community members are giving detailed accounts of their experiences. Issues of stigma and discrimination for people living with HIV remain an ongoing reality for many, and methodological choices can at times reinforce the experience of stigmatization. For example, surveys measuring HIV stigma and discrimination do not often allow people to provide additional details of their own experiences. For some communities, the acknowledgment of their members' experiences may be important, regardless of the specific research question. In these instances it may be necessary to make different methodological choices, or engage in multiple projects simultaneously.

While research studies need to be systematic and rigorous, they also need to remain flexible and specific to the context. Some researchers have pointed out that "[q]uestions about which methods are best suited to the situation need to be kept distinct from questions about whose opinions deserve more respect. The major pitfall is to accept compromises that would permit less than the highest quality research feasible" (Buchanan, Miller, & Wallerstein, 2007, p. 157).

While questions about methodological issues and decisions about methods have often been framed within the context of rigor, there are larger issues at stake as well. Community-based research has not only contributed to the democratization of knowledge, it has also opened up new and longstanding debates about multiple ways of knowing and the ownership of knowledge. While these debates are exciting and hold potential not only for the development of new knowledge, they also point to processes that are less predictable: processes in which ownership and power are always contested and new ways of doing things must be developed. Hence, for some people, community-based research is unpredictable, contingent, messy, complex, serendipitous, and challenging (Walton, Zraly, & Mugengana, 2014).

We agree that community-based research is always complex and at times also unpredictable and messy. Therefore, making methodological decisions given this context cannot be considered straightforward, definitive, or easy, particularly because methodological decisions also have to consider broader questions:

- Did the impetus for the research come from the community?
- Is attention being given to barriers to participation, with considerations of those who have been underrepresented in the past?
- Can the research facilitate collaboration between community participants and resources external to the community?
- Do community participants benefit from the research outcomes?
- Is there attention being given to, or an explicit agreement being made between, researchers and community participants with respect to ownership and dissemination of the research findings (Viswanathan et al., 2004)?

These questions point to the importance of integrating diverse methodologies and methods that respect both the limitations and possibilities of collaboration, ownership, resources, barriers, and ethics.

Political and Social Influences on Methodological Decisions

For some researchers (Savan et al., 2009), "the very questions we choose to ask, and the methods [and methodologies] we use to answer them are political" (p. 784). This recognition is perhaps accentuated in community-based research, where empowerment is a central tenant. With a primary goal of changing practice, policy, or behaviors to enhance social and environmental justice (Cargo & Mercer, 2008; Fletcher, 2003; Wright et al., 2010), participatory and community-based research approaches may be viewed by some researchers as biased and less objective. In fact, the primary focus of participatory research approaches is to understand the context (Wright et al., 2010), implicitly emphasizing the subjective nature of the research. We can see this in the Délı̨nę Uranium Research project, where the loss of many of the male elders was the initial impetus for the project. Some academics may perceive participant involvement in all aspects of the research as a threat to confidentiality, which in turn may compromise the support of some academics and ethics review boards for community-based research (Stanton, 2014). For example, when using a community participatory research approach, the line between the researchers and the participants becomes increasingly blurred. Chung and Lounsbury (2006) suggest that the blurring line between researcher and participant reflects an advanced stage of community participation referred to as "empowering co-investigation" (p. 2131). Guta, Nixon, and Wilson (2013b) also refer to the blurring of boundaries or "going native" (Stoecker, 2008) as positive features of community-based participatory research; the overlap between research, advocacy, and community development may in fact be a distinguishing feature of rigorous community-based research.

Francisco Ibáñez-Carrasco (2004), a Chilean-born Canadian AIDS activist and writer, makes an important argument when he discusses issues of desire and betrayal in relation to community-based research. He suggests that when using this approach, the "initial premise is that, as we engage with research, we inevitably desire someone/a cause/a way of making knowledge public—and we favor it—only to betray another" (p. 35). Within this argument is a recognition that community-based research is and must be seen as an ethical orientation to research; "that is, it is essential for researchers to demonstrate respect for community members" (Buchanan et al., 2007, p. 156).

The etymology of the word *respect*, while making visible the importance of relationships and regard, also holds a notion of *looking back* (Communitas 2001–2005). We wonder if this notion of looking back would mediate the inherent and unavoidable possibility of betrayal. Looking backward demands recognition of past places and times, but also connotes the presence of an anticipated future, or forward looking. As we engage in forward looking and anticipation of what might be, we must recognize that people and communities are always becoming; they are not fixed entities (Clandinin & Connelly, 2000). Considering this forward-looking notion makes betrayal a central issue, one that must also be weighed in terms of responsibilities and obligations of things yet to come. This was significant in the "Challenging Lifestyles" project Judy participated in, where interventions were reconsidered after team members analyzed the findings and engaged with other communities.

At the same time, Ibáñez-Carrasco (2004) also makes us think about the necessary intimacy of community-based research. As part of this intimacy, people close to the research—both academics and community members—are privileged to listen to, see, and witness experiences that perhaps they neither anticipated, nor wanted to know. Often it is in these moments that the fear of not knowing and the sense that everything has to be reported in research is most pronounced. This calls forth very particular questions about how we work collaboratively through these challenges and how, in partnership, we honor process and people, both individually and collectively.

In thinking about these questions, Vera recalls one of her recent experiences with the research ethics board. Vera, alongside academic colleagues and community members, submitted an ethics proposal in which the central goal was to understand the mitigation of the risk of sexual exploitation for young female children. The research was proposed within a community that experienced significant health, economic, and social disparities. The ethics board argued that without predicting what participants would share, researchers and community members would not be able to proceed with the proposed research. In these discussions it was clear that community members and researchers were willing to remain in ongoing conversations despite the possibility of not knowing, as well as be open to discussions about the possibilities to both silence and make knowledge visible. However, the ethics board members recommended using tools and measures to assess risk and risk mitigation rather than methodologies that asked girls who were potentially at risk to engage in research that involved life-history work. The research ethics board also raised questions about the community-based research approach and how we could work closely within the community while focusing on risk for sexual exploitation. While we recognized the potential for difficult stories to be told, as well as a risk of stigmatizing by focusing explicitly on risk for sexual exploitation, we also were very mindful that the community had come to work alongside the children and families and also had the most invested to address this issue. As we write this chapter, we find ourselves amid an appeals process of the ethics board decision at one university, while another university has given approval for this research to go ahead.

As we explore in chapter 6, the turn to ethical issues is central in community-based research and affects the political and social influences on methodological decisions. Some of these decisions are made within institutional structures such as ethics boards or funding agencies, neither of which know the community, the relationship between the community and the researchers, or the daily reality that might have shaped the experiences of the community. For others, community-based research plays a role in decolonizing research (Stanton, 2014), which is problematic for some ethics boards. The political and social dynamics also become evident as researchers and community members must answer questions about who is driving the research agenda and what is at stake within communities.

At first glance, these questions may appear disconnected from method-ological choices, but if taken seriously will affect the methodologies and methods used in research projects. Take, for example, a researcher's abil-ity to work with diverse methodologies and/or methods. Are individual researchers able to recognize that he/she may not be the best person to undertake the research? Are they willing to learn and engage with meth-odologies or methods that the community is interested in or feels are most appropriate? Would knowing multiple methodologies be feasible given the diverse and in-depth methodological approaches that exist? Or is the com-munity willing to seek new collaborators or connect with other researchers who may offer different methodological expertise? While these questions are not easy to answer, it is also important to consider that it takes addi-tional time and resources to develop partnerships and reciprocal rela-tionships, both of which are the foundation to building trustworthy and respectful collaborations essential to effective community-based research (Maiter et al., 2008).

Others have pointed out that research with geographically isolated communities is more difficult and that "[community-based research] principles are much easier to apply in proximal partnerships because they afford an environment where collaborative relationships can be developed and sustained" (Ritchie et al., 2013, p. 183). Do issues of proximity also affect methodological decisions? We argue that they do. Ethnographic or narrative methodologies, for example, are more chal-lenging to engage in with communities because research funding does not always take into consideration the increased cost of travel or the time spent within communities. In addition, few academics receive teaching release time to compensate them for the additional time required to carry out community-based research. At other times, logistical issues affect research projects. Vera still remembers conversations about where researchers would live in the community if they came for extended peri-ods of time during the Délı̨nę Uranium Research project. The choice of accommodation, for example, can influence how researchers are perceived within the community or with whom they hold alliances. Although this seems minor, it can not only influence the relationships but also affect important decisions that need to be made, such as: What if people disagree with findings? What if a potential outcome of the research is that programs may be cut off from funding sources? Who sanctions the research results?

Issues of relationships between community members and researchers, the dynamics of the relationship, and their different contexts affect all aspects of the research. Methodological decisions are affected by these fundamental relationships, as are the team compositions. Depending on the complexity of the research or the goal of the collaboration between communities and researchers, there may be a need to involve several researchers and community members or organizations, all of whom might contribute different philosophies and disciplinary knowledge. This adds another layer to the complexity and messiness of the research.

Rigor in Community-based Research

When using a community-based research approach, researchers must ensure that rigorous scientific methodologies are balanced with the adherence to the principles of community-based research. Despite this, we have found that occasionally funders and community organizations prioritize community involvement and partnerships over the scientific merit of research projects. Both components are critical. Meredith Minkler suggests that problems "may arise when community desires with respect to research design bump up against what outside researchers consider to be 'good science'" (2004, p. 692).

Although some may challenge the scientific merit of community-based research due to concerns about validity, reliability, and objectivity (Israel et al., 1998), the process of doing community-based research may actually enhance the rigor of the study. Recruitment and retention rates may be increased and measurement error may be decreased through the participation of non-academic partners in the design of instruments and the process of collecting data (Cargo & Mercer, 2008; Minkler, 2005). Similarly, knowledge dissemination is often strengthened and enriched during the community-based research process. Several authors (Cargo & Mercer, 2008; Macaulay et al., 1999; Minkler, 2005) suggest that jointly interpreting the data with the community increases internal and cultural validity of the findings, thereby enhancing the rigor of the study. These authors also argue that ethically sound participatory research may also promote ongoing capacity building, increased receptivity to future collaboration, and trust in the community partners. This was critical to the work of the Canadian Délı̨nę Uranium Team. Another beneficial outcome of participatory research is the refining of procedures for developing community advisory committees and (Macaulay et al., 1999) the strengthening of community ownership (Wallerstein & Duran, 2006). Christopher Fletcher, a Canadian researcher concerned with culture and diversity, argues that community-based research "can be conducted with methodological rigor and with contextual sensitivity" (2003, p. 37).

Although the benefits of using a community-based research approach are well documented, particularly for those familiar with the approach, Wright and colleagues (2010) argue that participatory approaches have "yet to achieve a clear scientific profile to serve as a basis for debating in what ways PHR [participatory health research] can make a unique contribution to building knowledge and theory" (p. 118). We concur with these authors that there is a need to define concepts such as objectivity, validity, and reliability in relation to participatory health research to evaluate the quality of participatory approaches. Wright and colleagues (2010) propose the formation of an international collaboration for participatory approaches to define participatory health research, identify its unique contributions, and develop standards for evaluation.

Christopher Fletcher (2003) developed the most comprehensive list of measures to assess rigor in community-based research (Table 4.1 on the next page lists some of Fletcher's most important criteria).

Though the full list of Fletcher's criteria is extensive and highlights issues of rigor, the perception that community-based research lacks methodological rigor and objectivity remains a central concern to those involved in the field. Many researchers have tried to develop or augment criteria over the years. Through their close work with key stakeholders in exploring practitioners' understanding of rigor, Kingsley and Chapman (2013) identify three themes, including obligations (which entail expectations and a sense of responsibility), representation, and a turn to action. They also identified relevance to practice as a key criterion for rigor. Others argue that "CBR [community-based research] reflects an emerging paradigm that denies the prior positivist notions of objectivity and neutrality of scientific research" (Hall, 1993, p. xiii).

Balazs and Morello-Frosch (2013), on the other hand, argue that community-based participatory research helps to improve the rigor, relevance, and reach of science. For these authors, community-based research is the practice and promotion of good science; hence, research using this

Table 4.1 List of Potential Criteria for Rigor

- Make the community the meeting ground for discussing the research
- Respect local political structures and processes
- Ensure transparency of research objectives
- Work out a reasonable and locally relevant timetable
- Listen closely
- Articulate research with local priorities and goals
- Use culturally appropriate research tools
- Be realistic about the significance and impact of research
- Establish mechanisms to deal with misunderstandings
- Give people an avenue to voice concerns throughout the research process
- Approach the relationship with the community participation as a commitment
- Work at communicating information in locally relevant terms
- Leave something behind in the community
- Document the research process
- Recognize local contributions
- Support local control over the research
- Provide appropriate compensation to participants and collaborators
- Establish how data will be controlled and managed

approach is rigorous. *Relevance* refers to consideration about whether the right question was asked, while *reach* examines the degree to which knowledge was disseminated and the process itself evaluated. Ultimately, when considering the question of rigor, researchers must ask, "How do we know if we are doing CBR well?" (Kingsley & Chapman, 2013, p. 551).

Several authors (Hall, 1993; Waterman, 1998) argue that rigor should be measured by how well the principles of community-based research are upheld, including attention to the moral responsibilities and ethical sensitivities in relation to people's lives. Springett, Wright, and Roche (2011) also call for a measure of quality that evaluates whether the standards of research are aligned with the core principles of community-based research. In all of these arguments, however, it is clear that the conceptualizations of rigor depend not only on the approach taken or methodologies chosen but also on the disciplinary and pragmatic foundations of the researchers and communities who engage in research. Interestingly, academics drive much of the debate about rigor. In our own work, the criteria developed by Aboriginal Cree scholar Verna Kirkness and colleague Ray Barnhard (2001) have been helpful and include respect, relevance, reciprocity, and responsibility. It has also been helpful for us to consider Marullo and colleagues' argument:

> Whereas traditional research relies on discipline-grounded theories and research methods to validate its questions, concepts, and methods, CBR requires two further criteria for validating research—the community's knowledge and experience as a critical prism through which meaning is constructed, and the utility of the findings for effecting social change. . . . Finally we note that as a consequence of CBR [community-based research] being grounded in the community context—carried out in conjunction with real-life, [including] ongoing, collective efforts to change social structures—the research and analysis is contingent on many more variables than can be controlled. (2003, p. 59)

Considering this, it is important to see methodological decisions in relation to epistemological and ontological understandings of community-based research; these decisions are not only pragmatic but also reflect commitments, responsibilities, and obligations. Reflecting on these responsibilities, we find it important to develop principles for research collaboration. These principles highlight the commitments and obligations by everyone involved and are discussed in greater detail in the next chapter.

5. Developing Principles for Research Collaboration

The increased complexity and interdisciplinary nature of most research programs requires that researchers develop principles for research collaboration early in the research process. Community-based research provides an excellent example of an approach to research that is complex, often interdisciplinary, and demands the engagement of partners from both community and academic settings. Principles for research collaboration are very specific principles that guide the conduct of the investigators, collaborators, and students involved in an individual research project or program. The principles may include: roles and responsibilities of each member of the research team; ethics and authorship guidelines; data storage; plans for capacity building, collaboration, and communication; and intellectual ownership principles. Several authors[1] recommend that academic and community researchers develop research agreements to outline the community-based research process and to ensure that ground rules are established should problems arise. Research agreements are also helpful to ensure that the local context is recognized and interventions are culturally supported (Wallerstein & Duran, 2006). In this chapter, we describe our experience with the development of research principles and provide examples of principles for research collaboration based on several research projects and programs.[2] To support this discussion, we review the literature in relation to research guidelines and complete the chapter with some reflections on the process of developing principles for research collaboration.

Essentials of Community-based Research by Vera Caine and Judy Mill, 61–68. © 2016 Left Coast Press, Inc. All rights reserved.

Background

In 2002, Judy Mill received funding from Health Canada for her first externally funded research project, "Challenging Lifestyles: Aboriginal Men and Women Living with HIV," which we discuss in detail in chapter 3. The research team included members from a small community organization that provided services to Aboriginal persons living with HIV and AIDS. As a novice researcher, Judy was very naive about the need to agree upon, at the beginning of the project, principles related to the management and ownership of data and the strategies for the dissemination of the findings. Although the team had discussions about the ethics of community-based research with Aboriginal communities, we did not develop principles for research collaboration. The lack of agreed-upon principles led to some tensions toward the end of the project, particularly in relation to authorship responsibilities. Judy led the writing of two manuscripts based on the findings from the "Challenging Lifestyles" project; however, the tensions were never openly discussed, and ongoing relationships with some members of the research team were compromised as a result.

Judy's first experience with the development of principles for research collaboration occurred in early 2003 when she received funding as the principal investigator for two Canadian Institute for Health Research (CIHR)–funded projects: "The Influence of Stigma on Access to Health Services by Persons with HIV Illness" and "The Diagnosis and Care of HIV Infection in Canadian Aboriginal Youth." Because both projects included the participation of Aboriginal individuals, Judy invited Randy Jackson, the research coordinator at the Canadian Aboriginal AIDS Network (CAAN), to join the research team. Randy became integral to the implementation of both projects and during early discussions of data ownership and authorship the team realized that it would be beneficial to develop a set of principles to guide their work. At first, Judy suggested that they develop a Memorandum of Understanding (MOU) to outline responsibilities. Advisors in the research office at Judy's university, however, did not feel that an MOU was an appropriate document[3] to outline this type of agreement for a research team; the team eventually agreed to develop principles for research collaboration. Principles were developed for each of the two projects and signed by representatives of CAAN and the other research team members. After this, Randy presented the principles for research collaboration at the Canadian Association for AIDS Research annual meeting (Jackson, Dixon, Thomas, & Zoccole, 2003) and developed a generic version of the principles in a CAAN fact sheet titled *Negotiating Ethical Agreements* (CAAN, 2010). Two of the research team members subsequently published a paper (Patterson, Jackson, & Edwards, 2006) on research ethics with Aboriginal communities based on their experiences with the stigma project.

Early in 2007, Judy Mill was part of a large interdisciplinary team that received funding from the Teasdale-Corti Global Health Research Initiative (GHRI) for a five-year program of research known as "Strengthening Nurses' Capacity for HIV Policy Development in Sub-Saharan Africa and the Caribbean." The GHRI, a collaborative partnership of CIHR, the Canadian International Development Agency, Health Canada, the International Development Research Centre, and the Public Health Agency of Canada, implemented the project using a participatory action research methodology. The purpose of the research program was to explore and promote nurses' involvement in HIV policy development in five low- and middle-income countries (LMICs) with a high HIV disease burden in sub-Saharan Africa (Kenya, Uganda, and South Africa) and the Caribbean (Jamaica and Barbados). The project team brought together researchers and decisionmakers from different disciplines and with divergent experience in research and publication practices. The team initially had three co-principal investigators (one each from Canada, sub-Saharan Africa, and the Caribbean) and 16 co-investigators representing researchers and decision-makers in the participating countries. Over the course of the first four years of the research program, the number of countries involved decreased.[4] However, the number of co-investigators increased to 25, and 16 collaborators, 7 graduate students, and 1 undergraduate student also participated in the research program. Capacity building was a major goal of the program (Edwards et al., 2007; Mill et al., 2014b) and opportunities for training were built into each phase of the research. The role of collaborator was specifically designed to foster capacity building: the collaborators and students contributed to the data collection and analysis while at the same time developing their research capacity.

The complexity of the overall research program, including the implementation of an intervention in the partner LMICs and the challenges related to the widespread locations of the research team members, necessitated the development of a set of principles to outline how the team would work together. The first version of the principles for research collaboration was developed and signed approximately one year after funding was received. A small working group chaired by Judy Mill developed the principles by virtual meetings. Once the working group had developed a draft of the principles for research collaboration, it was sent to the full research team for input. The project manager then coordinated signatures on the final version of the principles. The principles for research collaboration were revised and signed again in the fourth year of the project to add and remove collaborators and co-investigators and to clarify the role of project staff in relation to authorship. Although project staff were eligible to be authors on manuscripts, the research team felt that it was important to provide specific guidelines in terms of the number of manuscripts project staff could participate in and the need to complete their paid-work responsibilities prior to working on manuscripts. This was clarified in the final version of the principles for research collaboration.

In the next sections we provide a brief overview of the history of research and authorship guidelines. Based on what has been recommended by others, in combination with our own experiences, we suggest the key elements of and the process of developing principles for research collaboration.

Brief History of Research Guidelines

In the literature, there are few examples of guidelines about the research process. Although Israel and colleagues (1998) do not explicitly counsel the development of a research memorandum, they recommend "jointly developed operating norms" (p. 185) to facilitate the establishment of partnerships. A few years later, Fawcett and colleagues (2000) proposed that a Memorandum of Collaboration be developed at the outset of a research project to outline the roles and responsibilities of community partners, support organizations (including universities), and funding agencies. In 2003, Fletcher recommended the development of guidelines to ensure that Aboriginal communities maintained control over research agendas. Several authors[5] have recommended that community-based research teams develop MOUs to acknowledge the power differentials, outline the principles of engagement, and resolve difficult issues that might arise during the research. Ross and colleagues (2010) developed a framework to assist both academic and community researchers in identifying excellent partners, developing a work plan, planning the research design, and applying for funding, and highlighted issues related to recruitment, data collection, and analysis and dissemination. Despite these initiatives, researchers have not used guidelines to outline research relationships consistently until recently.

The development of authorship guidelines, on the other hand, is not a new endeavor. More than 30 years ago, Burman (1982) recommended that the criteria for authorship be negotiated in writing prior to and during a research study, but examples of what this written communication might include are difficult to find. In 1985, the International Committee of Medical Journal Editors (ICMJE) published *Guidelines on Authorship*, which has been widely referenced and continues to be a seminal document on authorship. The essence of these guidelines is that all authors must: (1) make a substantial contribution to the conception or design or analysis and interpretation of data or both; (2) be involved in writing and revising the manuscript for intellectual content; and (3) approve the final draft and be able to defend the published work. Huth (1986) supported and built on the ICMJE guidelines by outlining principles for different types of articles. In 1993, ICMJE updated the guidelines and reported that more than 500 biomedical journals were using the guidelines for the preparation of manuscripts. In 2009, ICMJE changed the first criteria in the guidelines to state that all authors must make "substantial contributions to conception *and* design, *acquisition of data*, or analysis and interpretation of data" (ICMJE, 2009; emphasis added). We suggest incorporating ICMJE's guidelines into the principles of research collaboration.

There are increasing opportunities for academic researchers and community partners to work together using a collaborative, community-based research approach; this increases the complexity of authorship decisions and the possibility of disagreement among team members. For example, members may disagree on the criteria for authorship and the order of authors on the statement of authorship (Burman, 1982). In a recent publication of the Council of Science Editors, Leash (2010) suggests that what is considered a contribution deserving of recognition through authorship may vary between departments, institutions, disciplines, and countries. Several authors (Grieger, 2005; Leash, 2010) have commented on the ethical issues related to the abuse of authorship. These authors highlight a variety of reasons for misconduct in authorship to occur among academics: increase in scientific research; pressure from academia; desire for prestige; tendency toward multidisciplinary, multisite research; and competition for funding. They suggest that the abuses of authorship may necessitate the explicit disclosure of authors' roles in the reported research.

Research projects and programs are inherently collaborative. However, collaboration among team members brings both benefits and costs to the research program (Katz & Martin, 1997). Benefits of research collaboration include shared resources, including knowledge, skills, and techniques; increased generation of new insights and perspectives; expanded research networks; and enhanced knowledge transfer (Katz & Martin, 1997). In a review of collaboration in HIV research, Onyancha and Ocholla (2007) report that research impact was almost three times higher in Kenya and two times higher in South Africa when the research was conducted through collaboration. Similarly, Ordonez-Matamoros, Cozzens, and Garcia (2009) found that for Colombian researchers, co-authoring with partners overseas contributes to team productivity and helps to ensure that the research addressed country-specific issues. Project leadership skills required to manage collaboration in research may be "as important to the success of the project as the research itself and [may] require as much 'work'" (Boyer, Orpin, & Walker, 2010, p. 107). The complexity of research programs, combined with the trends toward collaborative, interdisciplinary, and often large research teams, demand that research guidelines move beyond the traditional focus on authorship to include attention to issues such as ethical conduct, capacity building, data management, control of resources, and governance responsibilities of the research partners.

The development of research guidelines is particularly important for research programs when the partnerships between community and academic partners may be unequal due to differences in power, resources, and capacity. This is particularly important for community-based research with indigenous communities that may have been marginalized during previous research approaches (Fletcher, 2003; Macaulay et al., 1999) and international research programs in which formal management structures may be required (Katz & Martin, 1997). Therefore, to avoid power differentials, principles of research collaboration are needed to ensure that research programs are built on ethically sound principles. In a review of the benefits and challenges in collaborative HIV research in Africa, Cohen (2000) suggests that stresses and strains are part of collaborative research and often relate to issues of equity, including "access to financial resources and facilities, participation, transfer of technology, self-reliance, training opportunities, and credit" (p. 2155).

Developing Principles for Research Collaboration

Based on our experience in the development and implementation of principles for research collaboration, in combination with recommendations in the literature, we recommend that these principles include the following elements:

- Parties: Each member of the research team is listed, their affiliation highlighted, and the name of the research project or program stated.
- Purpose: A statement to confirm that the principles for research collaboration are to be used in conjunction with the relevant ethical guidelines (see below) for the conduct of research.
- Governance: The governance structure for the research project or program must be outlined to ensure that decision-making responsibilities are clearly articulated.
- Roles and Responsibilities: In this section, the roles and responsibilities of all members of the research team, including the principal investigator(s), co-investigators, project leads, graduate students, collaborators, interns, and research assistants, are outlined. These roles and responsibilities may include, but are not limited to: governance structure, preparation and submission of ethics applications, development of data collection tools, data collection and analysis, dissemination of findings, capacity-building activities, budgeting and financial oversight, preparing reports to funding organization, providing technical and scientific guidance, site visits, and participation in research team meetings.
- Records: Guidelines for the recordkeeping and storage of all data related to the project/program, during and beyond the period of funding, must be outlined in detail.
- Ethical Considerations: This section outlines the ethical guidelines to be followed in the research program, the process for signing confidentiality agreements, and the process for raising and dealing with ethical concerns that may arise during the research process. In Canada, *The Tri-Council Policy Statement: Ethical Conduct for Research Involving Humans* (Canadian Institutes of Health Research, Natural Sciences and Engineering Research Council of Canada, & Social Sciences and Humanities Research Council of Canada, 2010) must be followed.
- Capacity Building and Collaboration: The values and beliefs of the research team in relation to capacity building and collaboration should be outlined. These should be discussed initially during the development of the proposal, and on an ongoing basis following the receipt of funding.
- Ownership: The ownership of all of the intellectual components (e.g., proposal, data) of the program are discussed in this section. In addition, for research involving Indigenous communities, specific principles related to ownership, control, access, and possession (see Schnarch, 2004) must be considered.
- Communication: Responsibilities for communication of relevant administrative decisions (e.g., meeting dates, contract decisions, and changes to ethics protocols) are outlined in this section.
- Duration and Amendments: It is important to detail the time period when the principles of research collaboration will be in effect and outline the procedure for review and amendment. In addition, it is important to outline how decisions related to data access, secondary data analysis, and authorship will be made in the post-funding period. This is critical because data analysis and research dissemination are typically not complete when the funding ends.

- Authorship: Criteria for authorship on data from the project/program are outlined in this section. In addition, the protocol for the resolution of conflict in relation to authorship is reviewed.
- Signatures: The final section includes the name, date, and signature of each member of the research team.

In addition to these elements, Macaulay and colleagues (1999) suggest that research agreements should include statements about the degree and types of confidentiality and the process for resolving disagreements.

Looking Back and Moving Forward

Judy's early experience in the development of principles of research collaboration with Aboriginal community partners, in combination with her recent experiences in the use of principles of research collaboration for an international research program, have led her to become a firm promoter of principles of research collaboration for all projects and programs of research. On several occasions the "Strengthening Nurses' Capacity" team referred to their principles of research collaboration to ensure that decision-making was fair and consistent. Rules governing research partnerships should be established early in the research process (Jones & Wells, 2007) to provide structure, while at the same ensuring flexibility to accommodate unanticipated change and maximize the sustainability of partnerships (Israel et al., 2006, 2008). Memorandums of Understanding ensure that the expectations of all parties are delineated and the terms of the agreement are outlined (Ross et al., 2010).

The current nature of research, including interdisciplinary, large teams that may be based in communities and academia and situated in different regions of the world, has increased the complexity of research and the potential for power differentials. A principles for research collaboration agreement will help to equitably protect all members of the research team by ensuring that the principles guiding the conduct of the investigators, collaborators, and students are agreed upon in advance. We argue that when beginning a community-based research project or program, the development of principles for research collaboration is critical to the success of the research partnership.

In addition to the development of principles for research collaboration, researchers contemplating the use of community-based research must become familiar with the ethical challenges that accompany this approach and the strategies that may be used to mitigate these challenges. We explore these in depth in the next chapter.

Section III
Contexts and Challenges

6. Raising Ethical Questions

Despite the many benefits that accrue when using a community-based research approach, researchers contemplating community-based research must consider the ethical challenges inherent to the approach and use appropriate strategies to overcome these challenges. This is critical to ensure community-based research is ethical. Mikesell, Bromley, and Khodyakov (2013) highlight several characteristics of ethical community-based research: collaboration with communities, engaging in research that is beneficial to the community, and allowing the community to control the research process. The characteristics of ethical community-based research are very similar to the principles of community-based research, emphasizing the need for rigorous community-based research that is aligned with these characteristics.

Following a systematic review to explore ethics in community-based health research, Mikesell and colleagues (2013) also identify a number of ethical challenges: managing dual roles as community members and researchers; insider-outsider tensions; working with ethics review boards; investment of time; resource and funding challenges; the cyclical, iterative

Essentials of Community-based Research by Vera Caine and Judy Mill, 69–80. © 2016 Left Coast Press, Inc. All rights reserved.

nature of community-based research; community representation, protection, and commitment; and dissemination of findings. Minkler (2004) highlights several very similar challenges related to community-based participatory research and provides case studies to highlight each of them: (1) ensuring a true community-driven agenda; (2) acknowledging the insider-outsider tension that may arise due to differences in race, power, time, and rewards; (3) recognizing racial and cultural issues; (4) considering the limits of participation; and (5) dealing with issues related to the ownership and dissemination of the findings. In this chapter we explore several of these challenges and strategies to overcome them. In addition, we highlight some of the ethical challenges related to the rigor of community-based research and conclude with a general discussion of strategies to ensure ethical community-based research.

Managing Dual Roles

Community-based research challenges academic researchers to broaden their traditional academic framework to consider the implications of research with community partners (Shore et al., 2008). For example, the close relationships that develop with both participants and community research partners are often uncomfortable from the perspective of academics. In describing her work with communities, Meiners (2004) comments that "activism moves me into kinds of relationships that academia discourages, prohibits, and actively disqualifies" (p. 175). During the "Challenging Lifestyles" project (Mill et al., 2007), which Judy led, Douglas, one of the research participants, arrived unexpectedly and uninvited at one of the Community Advisory Committee meetings. At first Judy was quite uncomfortable about this because from an academic perspective, there is no provision in the ethical approval for research participants to change roles. Despite this, one of the community research members reassured Judy that this fluidity in roles is quite common and appropriate in community-based research. The participant was very keen to join the Community Advisory Committee to participate in the planning and dissemination of the research findings. He did this in a very professional manner; after this experience, he turned his life around, wrote a book about his life experiences, and volunteered on several HIV community boards. The tension that this incident initially caused for Judy was alleviated when she listened to the advice of her community partner. This experience was a genuinely positive one for Douglas and was achieved by trusting and listening to community partners.

Insider–Outsider Tensions

Developing authentic relationships and maintaining partnerships can be challenging. Tensions may develop between the *outside* academic researcher and the *inside* community partner or between research team members with more power and those with less. For example, how do team members determine allegiance when tension is apparent between one or more of the community partners? During our mentorship project (Mill et al., 2014a), we became aware of tensions between David, one of our advisory committee members, and the community agencies that he was involved with or received service from. We had several discussions about how to resolve this conflict and particularly how to deal with the tension when the conflicting team members were at the same table. Ultimately we dealt with this situation by talking with the respective parties individually rather than during the advisory committee meeting.

The issue of race and privilege is another potential tension that may surface when using a community-based research approach. Chavez, Duran, Baker, Avila, and Wallerstein (2008) use a dancing metaphor to highlight the need for academic and community researchers to "complement each other's steps, sometimes leading, sometimes following" (p. 91) and also to reflect on their mistakes when they are made. These authors argue that power imbalances between research team members may obstruct the development of trust required to build relationships in community-based research. The issue of power, and the potential for unequal power, is ever present in community-based research projects and must be continuously considered during the implementation process.

Working with Ethics Review Boards

In the past, a primary concern of ethics review boards was to ensure that the research was *objective* and that the participants or subjects remained passive participants in the research process. A community-based research approach however, requires that the *research subjects* are viewed as equitable community partners who contribute unique strengths to the process (Shore et al., 2008), thereby making the distinction between objectivity and subjectivity blurry (Flicker et al., 2008b). Traditionally, active community involvement in research was discouraged and the benefits of research to communities were not considered. Research ethics reviews must be able to provide a blended review to assess the risk to research participation at both the individual and community levels.[1] Additional ethical considerations are required to ensure that both perspectives are considered. These considerations include attention to, and respect for, community autonomy, social and community justice, and community beneficence (Mikesell et al., 2013). Some communities recently developed their own process for the ethical review of research projects (Shore et al., 2008) that may add another dimension to the process of launching research.

Guta and colleagues (2013b) completed a review of North American ethics boards to examine protocols that use a community-engaged approach to research, particularly in relation to the phenomenon of *ethics creep*. These authors define "ethics creep" as the increasing bureaucratization and requirements of ethics review boards prior to approving research. However, they uncovered few examples of this phenomenon, and questioned whether concerns about ethics creep might be diverting attention from the increasing types of research methodologies, ethics review procedures, structures of ethics review boards, and the realities of institutional research cultures. The authors conclude that "ethics review sits at the crossroads of power/knowledge" (p. 308) and argue that the growing pressure on academics to produce more evidence while working more closely with communities increases the potential for harm to individuals and communities.

We along with colleagues (Mill et al., 2014a) recently completed a research project that focuses on the mentorship of nurses providing HIV care and highlights the challenges related to obtaining multiple approvals. Due to the involvement of community and academic researchers, community-based organizations, and clinical agencies, 16 ethics and administrative approvals were required to implement the research. The Canadian Institutes of Health Research [CIHR]'s *Tri-Council Policy Statement on Ethics in Human Research* (CIHR et al., 2010) is based on the principles of respect, welfare, and justice and helps to ameliorate some of the complex issues that arise in community-based research. In addition, there is a section in these guidelines that provides specific principles for the conduct of research with Aboriginal communities (refer to chapter 8 in this book for further details).

Academic and community partners may have differing opinions about the need for, and value of, research ethics boards. Communities are sometimes puzzled by the role of university ethics boards and feel that they should possess the sole decision-making power over research projects in their communities. This is particularly common when working with Indigenous community partners. Flicker and colleagues (2007) reviewed the forms and guidelines for 30 ethics review boards in North America and report that the documents portray an overwhelmingly biomedical perspective, focused on protecting the individual, and reflect the perception that academic researchers have the exclusive right to produce and disseminate knowledge. These researchers found that ethics review documents rarely reflect the principles of community-based research and make the following recommendations to enhance the rigor of community-based research: ethics review boards should be provided with training opportunities; community-based research projects should provide terms of reference signed by all research partners; and community-based research projects should outline their decision-making process.

One of the unique challenges faced by academic research ethics boards is that they may not understand the role and contribution of advisory committees, an important feature of community-based research (van de Sande & Schwartz, 2011). In addition, the community-based research approach may result in processes unfamiliar to academic research ethics boards: the sharing of power may result in more than one principal investigator, it may be difficult to guarantee anonymity and confidentiality, the methodology may change during the research, and the community may want to store some of the raw data (van de Sande & Schwartz, 2011). For example, the roles of the individuals involved may change during the research process, thereby altering the methodology agreed upon at the beginning of the project. This role variability is highlighted in the previous section of this chapter ("Managing Dual Roles") in the story about Douglas. DeSantis (2014) refers to the movement of individuals in and out of research activities in community-based research as the process of inclusion/exclusion.

From an academic perspective, the nature of community-based research demands that permission for the research must be vetted not only by university ethics boards, but also by ethics boards in communities (Shore et al., 2008). When possible, it is advantageous to ask the community partners to suggest which ethics review board will review the proposed research. In addition, administrative approval to conduct the research must be obtained from each partner organization in the community. The process of seeking administrative approval can contribute to the time required to complete the study, and at times the researcher may seek permission from, and collaborate with, a partner that does not represent the interests of the community (Macaulay et al., 1999).

In the past, university ethics boards were reticent to allow researchers to give tobacco as a gift; however, this hesitation has decreased in recent years as ethics boards have come to understand the rationale behind this practice. When conducting research with Indigenous individuals and communities in Canada, tobacco is often used as a gift to elders who are asked to say a prayer to guide a meeting or to participate throughout the research project. This protocol is dependent on where the research takes place and who is asked to participate. Regardless, the researcher should consult with an Indigenous community member to determine the local practice in relation to gifts and should build this into the application of the ethics review board.

Investment of Time

The increased time required to do community-based research is an ever-present and often challenging issue. This challenge is coupled with the sometimes-erroneous attitudes of members of the academic community toward this approach to research. Developing trusting relationships, engaging community members, and incorporating capacity-building opportunities for team members takes more time than traditional approaches to research. Vera is reminded of the Délı̨nę Uranium Research project, where it took several years to build the capacity for people to write and translate interviews and documents in the North Slavey language. As a result of the additional time required, academic researchers may be tempted to revert to more traditional approaches to research (Stanton, 2014). Stanton suggests that if the additional time required to carry out community-based research is not allowed for, it may actually be seen as disrespectful to Indigenous individuals and communities. Stoecker (2008) explores the notion of whether academics are irrelevant in community-based research. He argues that to facilitate community-controlled knowledge and encourage social change, academics typically adopt the role of initiator, consultant, or collaborator when engaged in community-based research. In addition, academics must be comfortable admitting how much they don't know and how much they can learn from the community.

The Cyclical, Iterative Nature of Community-based Research

Community-based research cannot be carried out using a prescriptive approach that is appropriate for all types of research in all contexts. Therefore, community-based research researchers must be creative, adaptive, and willing to negotiate the methodology, including the data collection process, the research sites, and the dissemination strategies. This approach often requires a very fine balance between the approved research protocol, the community needs, and the scientific rigor of the study. Strickland (2006) highlights the importance of understanding the ebb and flow of the community when working with Indigenous partners. For example, she found that by scheduling meetings at convenient times and providing food and other incentives, she was able to encourage participation in meetings.

Community and academic partners may have different perspectives on the outcomes of the research and dissenting opinions about the emphasis to place on the tasks versus the process of the research (Israel et al., 1998). Researchers must be sensitive to this challenge and willing to make adjustments to the research protocols to accommodate these differences. Following our mentorship project, the community members of the research team were particularly interested in writing about the process of doing the research. To ensure that the needs and wishes of all partners are met, we advocate the preparation of principles for research collaboration (see chapter 5) at the outset of the research project.

Resource and Funding Challenges

Although there is growing support for community-based research from academics (Minkler & Wallerstein, 2008) and funding agencies (e.g., National Institutes of Health [USA] and Canadian Institutes for Health Research, Community-based Research [Canada]), current funding constraints in many North American universities may make it very difficult to secure the time and money required to develop successful community-based research partnerships. As a result of this challenge, some faculties and universities have an implicit bias toward research that is quicker and less *messy*. Many faculty members are not rewarded for their efforts at community-engaged scholarship, and therefore the reward for conducting community-based research must be more intrinsic and personal. Stoecker (2008) argues that the reward system in universities may actually discourage the collaboration required in community-based research. In addition, the tendency to produce papers with multiple authors that is common with community-based approaches may lead some academics to prefer more traditional approaches to research. Several authors (Burke et al., 2013; MacLean et al., 2009) highlight the need for academic researchers to be trained in community-based research approaches and argue that policies that support community-based research are required within universities.

Historically, the payment of individuals and organizations has been considered coercive in the research process. However, the payment of individuals for his/her time working with the researchers has become the standard and preferred practice when using a community-based research approach. In the Déline Uranium Research project, community members were provided with paid employment whenever possible. Flicker and colleagues (2007) reiterate the importance of valuing and compensating community members for their time. In the research we have conducted, the community participants often do not have paid employment; therefore, the payment for their time acknowledges their substantial expertise and contribution to the project. Similarly we have encouraged individuals who work in community-based organizations to accept payment for their participation, even when participating on paid time, recognizing that their participation has taken place on organizational time. In this case we suggest that the individual donate the payment to their organization. This is important, particularly when the positions community members hold do not include research activities. Typically the employee has had to work late before or after the research meetings to meet their community-based organization commitments. Government-paid representatives, on the other hand, are often unable to accept honoraria or payment for their participation in a research project. In all cases, individuals and communities must be paid for expenses related to participating in the research including travel, child care, and meal costs (Minkler et al., 2003).

In a survey of Canadian researchers conducting community-based research, Flicker and colleagues (2008b) highlight insufficient funding as an impediment to adopting a community approach to research. The funding challenges were related to the inability to hire staff to support the research, the inflexibility of funders related to the requirements of doing community-based research, and the need to pay cash to some research team members who did not have a credit card or were living in poverty. On several occasions we recall funding research expenses from our own pocket, picking up and driving community researchers to meetings, or driving to a hotel late at night to provide a credit card because a community elder did not have one. DeSantis (2014) reminds us that funding agencies will often fund the *research* component of community-based research, but will seldom fund the advocacy element of the partnership.

Plumb and colleagues (2004) also point out that funding may not cover the time required to establish authentic partnerships with communities and pay community collaborators. These authors highlight the need for funding agencies to evaluate and provide funding for both the scientific rigor and community collaboration of research. In addition, in an evaluation of community research partnerships, community research partners often found the reviews provided by funding review panels overly "harsh" (Plumb et al., 2004, p. 436), sometimes discouraging the community organization from reapplying for funding. These authors suggest that community organizations may not understand the culture, policies, and practices of both funders and academic organizations.

Dissemination of Findings

When negotiating community-based research, the final products of the research are often different depending on the viewpoint of the partner. Differences in perspectives, assumptions, values, priorities, and language may lead to conflicts among research team members (Flicker et al., 2007; Israel et al., 1998). For example, despite the reliance by academic researchers on peer-reviewed publications, other products such as final reports, presentations, pamphlets, artwork, websites, and video clips may be preferred by community partners to disseminate research.

Despite the increased likelihood that findings from community-based research will be disseminated using nontraditional approaches, funders do not typically accommodate these strategies (Flicker et al., 2007; Martz & Bacsu, 2014), and academic institutions may place a lower value on these approaches compared with peer-reviewed publications (MacLean et al., 2009). In addition, the collaborative nature of community-based research often means that many research reports, publications, and other products of research are coauthored (Nyden, 2003). This may be a significant departure from traditional, discipline-specific dissemination strategies. Community partners and organizations are often most interested in preparing a final report, while academic researchers are commonly valued by their colleagues and measured by academic review boards based on their peer-reviewed publications. How do the research partners decide which and in what order the various dissemination tools will be used? We suggest that it depends on the research team and the research findings. For example, in one of our research projects that focused on HIV testing in Aboriginal youth (Mill et al., 2008), in addition to traditional peer-reviewed publications, the team prepared a pamphlet for youth about HIV testing that was distributed by the community-based partner organizations. One key outcome for the Délı̨nę Uranium Research project was the production of a dual-language book written in both English and North Slavey that included historical records and the voices of community members.

Ensuring Ethical Community-based Research

Several authors highlight strategies to overcome challenges and ensure that research using a community-based research approach is ethically sound. We agree with several authors (Mikesell et al., 2013; van de Sande & Schwartz, 2011) that the involvement of community members must occur early and in all stages of the research, from the development of the problem to the dissemination of the findings, for high-quality scholarship to take place. A community-based participatory approach implies that community members are equal partners in the research (Chung & Lounsbury, 2006) and the involvement and knowledge of community and lay members are maximized throughout the process (Cargo & Mercer, 2008). Ann Macaulay, who has worked extensively with the Mohawk community of Kahnawake in central Canada, and colleagues (1999) stress the importance of mutual respect and trust during the establishment of partnerships between academic and community researchers in the participatory research process. It takes time to establish trust, and because of differences in the backgrounds, areas of expertise, and organizational affiliations of the team members, trust and respect should never be taken for granted. Trust in academic researchers is enhanced when a respected community member facilitates the entry of the academic into the community (Martz & Bacsu, 2014).

Although ethics review boards are necessary to ensure that individuals are protected from harm during the research process, community review boards may be required to ensure the interests of the community are considered and respected (Mikesell et al., 2013). The education of ethics review board members, the development of an evaluation framework to ensure rigorous community-based research, and preparation of a research agreement (see chapter 5) to outline the expectations of team members are also recommended to ensure ethical community-based research (Mikesell et al., 2013). Macaulay and Nutting (2006) argue that the development of a research agreement can strengthen the partnership and lead to more rigorous research. Engaging with community members in community-based research also helps to keep academic researchers accountable to the focus of the research. For example, David was a major driving force in keeping us accountable to people living with HIV by ensuring that our research was congruent with the Greater Involvement of People Living with AIDS (GIPA) principles and achieved the desired outcomes.

Benatar and Singer (2010) argue that research in resource-poor countries must acknowledge the linkages between research ethics, health, and social justice. These authors suggest that in addition to the production of new knowledge and the building of capacity in local researchers, academic researchers must ensure that the outcomes of research benefit the health and well-being of the community they are working with when conducting international research. This principle could also be applied more generally to community-based research because it is often undertaken with individuals and communities that live with inequities. Therefore, to ensure that research positively influences the health of resource-poor communities, we concur with Benatar and Singer (2010) that researchers must seek robust engagement with communities, understand local conditions, and establish trusting relationships. This approach to research is congruent with the principles of community-based research in any setting.

Although we have tried to illuminate many of the ethical questions related to community-based research and to suggest some appropriate interventions, some questions remain that a researcher may face and feel unsure about answering. See the box on the next page for some examples.

We hope that the challenges we discuss here will assist community-based researchers in designing research that is ethically sound. Another key consideration in the process of implementing community-based research is authentic partnership and capacity building with community partners. In fact, we believe that capacity building is a key feature of ethical research with communities. In the next chapter, we explore the concept of capacity building as it relates to community-based research, including factors such as readiness that are essential to building and sustaining capacity.

Ongoing Questions

It is standard practice for academic researchers to ensure that an ethics review board reviews all research. The nature of community-based research, however, begs the question of whether it is ethical for academic researchers to be involved with community research in the preliminary fieldwork stage that has *not* received ethical approval. During preliminary fieldwork, researchers develop research questions, make methodological choices, and often initiate and/or affirm relationships (Caine, Davison, & Stewart, 2009).

Another question that may come up with community-based research is what the ethical implications are when the communities do not approve of a research project. For example, if there is an Ebola outbreak spreading in Africa, is it appropriate for researchers to conduct research on interventions, including new vaccines and viral strains, if the community members and leadership do not support the project? Are there times when a broader understanding of *global* community needs take precedence over the *local* community needs?

7. Considering Capacity

Traditional research projects often fail to give back to, and build capacity within, individuals and communities (Flicker et al., 2007). Much like in the Délı̨nę Uranium Research project, the involvement of community members is central to community-based research and is an empowering process that builds capacity (Guta, Flicker, & Roche, 2013a; Wright et al., 2010). We argue that building capacity among research partners is one of the hallmarks of rigorous, ethical research. Although there is evidence to suggest that participatory approaches foster capacity building, there have been limited attempts to conceptualize capacity building in relation to empowerment and ownership (Cargo & Mercer, 2008).

Capacity building in community-based research refers to the development of skills and expertise at both the individual and organizational levels (Minkler, 2004). We concur with Vogel's (2011) definition of research capacity building as "a context specific, dynamic process that goes beyond a technical or value-neutral transfer of skills" (p. 12). Many authors have demonstrated strong commitments to capacity building in community-based research with youth (Flicker et al., 2008c), women (Mill et al., 2012), and nurses (Mill et al., 2014a). Despite the positive outcomes in a survey that explored the status of community-based research in Canada, Flicker and colleagues (2008b) report that research projects that focus on marginalized communities find it particularly challenging to build the capacity of community members to become co-researchers. Mill and colleagues (2014b) also report several challenges related to the development of capacity among nurses in low- and middle-income countries. Although capacity building is generally considered a positive outcome of

Essentials of Community-based Research by Vera Caine and Judy Mill, 81–87. © 2016 Left Coast Press, Inc. All rights reserved.

community-based research, Guta and colleagues (2013a) remind us of the dangers of capacity building when the goals are not congruent with those of the individuals involved.

In this chapter, we focus on capacity building as an essential and critical component of community-based research. We highlight the need for cultural humility as foundational to the development of capacity. In addition, we explore individual and organizational readiness as they relate to successful capacity building. Structures in universities, community organizations, and funding agencies that promote or inhibit capacity building are critical to organizational readiness. Finally, we discuss the importance of ongoing commitment to the sustainability of capacity that is developed.

Cultural Humility

The need to ensure that both the context and the culture of communities are considered and respected is foundational to capacity building and critical to the success of community-based research. This concept has been referred to as *cultural safety* by some (Harrowing, Mill, Spiers, Kulig, & Kipp, 2010) and *cultural competence* by others. The concept of *cultural humility* was described and advocated almost two decades ago (Tervalon & Murray-Garcia, 1998); however, it has only recently been advocated by a number of authors[1] as a more appropriate and comprehensive concept than cultural competence to ensure a deep understanding of culture. Some authors (Fisher-Borne, Montana Cain, & Martin, 2015; Ross, 2010) critique the concept of cultural competence for several reasons: it does not take into account structural factors that influence individuals' experiences; there is limited emphasis on a critical self-awareness of culture; and racial identity is often conflated with culture. Fisher-Borne and colleagues (2014) argue that cultural humility offers greater promise as a conceptual framework for social work because it acknowledges the dynamic nature of culture, advocates for providers' self-awareness of power differentials between themselves and clients, and challenges individuals and institutions to tackle inequities. Furthermore, they argue that achieving cultural humility is "an ongoing process without a finite endpoint" (p. 7) that incorporates accountability at both the individual and institutional levels. The principles of cultural humility are highly relevant to understanding culture and context in the process of conducting community-based research.

Various researchers advocate for the need for research that acknowledges the importance of culture when conducting international research (Harrowing et al., 2010; Mill & Ogilvie, 2002). By doing so, researchers help to ensure the research is ethical. Harrowing and colleagues (2010) suggest that researchers who engage in global research must give careful consideration to "the cultural and social context and values of the proposed setting in order to situate the research within the appropriate ethical framework" (p. 70). Similarly, Mill and Ogilvie (2002) argue that in addition to adhering to universal ethical principles for the protection of human participants, international research must also acknowledge the ethical standards related to the cultural environment and the institutional setting. Although these authors focus on international research, we support the argument that attention to cultural context in all research is critical to ethically sound research and is a prerequisite to developing capacity.

Readiness

A question that many researchers ask is whether *all* communities are able and ready to lead community-based research projects. Capacity building is dependent on the stage of readiness (Cargo & Mercer, 2008); however, the readiness and capacity of partners is an ongoing challenge. Readiness depends on the strengths, expertise, and capacity of the community. Similarly, researchers must evaluate the readiness of academic partners to embrace a community-based research approach. Readiness to engage in community-based research can be assessed from both an individual and community perspective.

Individual Readiness

Individual readiness to engage in community-based research is influenced by a number of factors among community members. Opportunities for research training, the motivation to participate in research, and adequate time to participate in research are all factors that contribute to individual readiness. In considering individual readiness to embrace community-based research and develop capacity, a prior working relationship with a community organization is a factor that can facilitate the development of collaborative relationships (Israel et al., 1998), thereby enhancing individual readiness.

Stoecker (2008) stresses the importance of capacity building and describes a community-based research project that was unsuccessful because the community members had not been adequately trained to conduct interviews. Judy Mill faced similar challenges with the conduct of qualitative interviews during a large research program (Mill et al., 2014b) to explore nurses' involvement with HIV policy in sub-Saharan Africa and the Caribbean. The research program, using 13 qualitative tools, was launched without adequately exploring the prior opportunities for the research assistants to receive training in the conduct of in-depth interviews. The volume of the qualitative data, combined with the relatively few experienced qualitative researchers, made it difficult to provide timely feedback to the research assistants on the quality of the interview data. This resulted, particularly early in the data collection process, in some research assistants exploring the research questions in a superficial manner.

Organizational Readiness

Organizational readiness refers to the capacity and willingness of community, academic and funding organizations to participate in research. Public expectations related to accountability have resulted in some nonprofit organizations feeling forced to engage in research to justify their work (Flicker, 2008) or being inadequately compensated with the resources (both time and money) needed to participate in research (Flicker et al., 2008c). This reality is magnified by the expectation of funders that academic researchers must engage with community partners, and has resulted in some community organizations leading research when they lack the interest and expertise to do so. Wallerstein and Duran (2006) suggest that sometimes community partners join research teams to access funds rather than due to their interest in the research questions. In the Délı̨nę Uranium Research project, the community, by taking local control, was also able to develop ongoing plans for capacity building. Researchers who engaged with the community were asked to provide workshops and training.

Structures in universities and community organizations may also present challenges to the implementation of community-based research (Strickland, 2006) and affect organizational readiness to support capacity building. For example, faculty evaluation and promotion committees in universities may not place high value on research that takes more time than traditional methods do and results in publications with multiple academic and community partners (Strickland, 2006). In addition, some academic researchers may view community-based research as a threat because it is based on the principle of shared power and knowledge, thus challenging the traditional approach to who defines the problem, how the research is approached, and how the research outcomes are used (Nyden, 2003). Nyden (2003) argues that "the traditional culture of research also worships the theoretical and devalues the practical" (p. 577) and views community-based research as political, potentially resulting in biased research. This is particularly true in discipline-specific and professional faculties that have traditionally defined the research agenda (Nyden, 2003). Similarly, funding agencies may not provide funding that adequately covers the time involved to develop and maintain partnerships before and between research projects (Strickland, 2006). Funders typically have strict guidelines about who can hold funds and how funds can be spent, often impeding the active involvement of communities in the research.

Nyden (2003) suggests several incentives for academics to challenge the status quo and participate in community-based, participatory research. To mitigate the challenges that academic researchers experience when carrying out community-based research, he suggests that universities modify faculty tenure and promotion guidelines to encourage and reward community-based research, encourage team approaches and networks to facilitate community-based research, develop rigorous measures to evaluate community-based research, and use ethics boards to ensure that in addition to individual protection, the benefits for communities are considered. In addition, both universities and funding agencies must ensure that there are sufficient resources for community-based research.

Readiness in funding organizations must be assessed prior to initiating community-based research. Although there is increased funding and support for community-based research (Minkler et al., 2003), there is still more work to be done to promote the success and sustainability of research with communities. Several authors (Macaulay & Nutting, 2006; Minkler et al., 2003) argue that funding agencies have a role to play in helping to build communities, either directly or through an intermediary organization, to ensure there is sufficient time to build the authentic relationships required to develop capacity. These authors argue that a community-based research approach must enable researchers in low-income communities to develop the capacity to become equitable research partners. This is similar to the argument by Benatar and Singer (2010) that research programs in resource-poor countries have an ethical obligation to contribute to building the capacity and improving the health of participants who are part of the research. Funding is required to ensure that communities have the capacity to review, participate in, and ultimately manage community-based research projects (Minkler, 2004; Shore et al., 2008).

Sustainability: Ongoing Commitment

Community-based research is a long-term process that requires sustained commitment to the approach (Israel et al., 2008). As discussed in chapter 2, partnership synergy is critical to the success and sustainability of the collaborations required to do community-based research. Cargo and Mercer (2008) advocate incorporating mechanisms into the design of community-based research to sustain the research partnerships. Based on their experience with partnership synergy research, Lasker and Weiss (2003) remind us that the ability of partners to understand health issues and sustain interventions is dependent not only on who and how community stakeholders are involved but also on the leadership of the partnership. Similarly, London (2007) points out that when one is doing community-based research with youth, particularly in low-income communities, long-term community capacity may be enhanced through networks rather than a single organization.

The building of trust to authentically engage with participants means that community-based research demands an ongoing commitment of all members of the research team. This level of commitment is typically contrary to the training academics receive about the research process. In a recent large, multidisciplinary team of researchers, community members, and decision-makers from Canada and four low- and middle-income countries (Mill et al., 2014b), some of the Canadian team members never met any of the low- and middle-income countries' team members. Although the focus of the training and capacity building opportunities was primarily the low- and middle-income countries' team members, this aspect of the design made it very challenging to develop the trust, build the relationships, and sustain the commitment required by all team members to implement the participatory action research program across wide a geographical area.

Israel and colleagues (2006) explore factors that contribute to the sustainability of community-based research. These authors suggest that factors that facilitate the continuation of community-based research partnerships include the sustainability of the relationships and commitments among partners; the knowledge, capacity, and values generated from the research; and the funding, staff, and programs that have been developed. Although community-based research can be highly successful in a wide variety of contexts, funding agencies rarely provide sufficient funding to sustain the partnerships and relationships beyond the dissemination phase (Cargo & Mercer, 2008; Flicker et al., 2007). Youth participants in Flicker's (2008) study expressed frustration with securing funding to sustain the community-based research project in which they had participated. Similarly, London (2007) reminds us that community research with youth must take a long-term perspective, and that researchers must consider the capacity of organizations to support the meaningful involvement of youth over time.

The need to incorporate strategies to build the capacity of all research team members is fundamental to the conduct of community-based research. A variety of factors often make the sustainability of the partnerships developed during community-based research projects very challenging. These include research funding that does not extend past the dissemination stage, tenure and promotion guidelines that do not reward involvement in community-based research, and the increased time required to use a community-based research approach. This in turn may limit the depth and quality of capacity building opportunities that are available, particularly for community members. Researchers who use community-based research approaches must ensure that the development of capacity is built into the design of community-based research projects and advocate for strategies to overcome barriers to capacity building.

Capacity building in community-based research is foundational to ensure that communities are able to take ownership in the planning and implementation of research. In the next chapter, Randy Jackson and Renée Masching use their extensive experience to highlight the strengths and challenges of using community-based research with Aboriginal communities in Canada. Their insights raise questions and offer solutions to the issues that surface in the conduct of community-based research with diverse communities.

8. Working with Diverse Populations: A Focus on Aboriginal Communities in Canada

Randy Jackson and Renée Masching

Questions about diverse populations are frequently raised in community-based research. For Indigenous peoples, community-based research has been a welcomed approach, as it holds promise for affirming the principles of self-determination in the research process. Particularly in Canada, community-based research approaches support the values that Aboriginal[1] peoples bring to this work. These values "revolve around [issues of] trust, respect, self-determination, mutuality of interests, perspective taking, full participation, reciprocity, collective benefit, and long-term commitment" (Manson et al., 2004, p. 73S). From our experiences working with the Canadian Aboriginal AIDS Network (CAAN), community-based research is a meaningful and robust approach that has become, along with Indigenous and decolonizing methodologies, the foundation for our research.

Essentials of Community-based Research by Vera Caine and Judy Mill, 89–108. © 2016 Left Coast Press, Inc. All rights reserved.

This chapter highlights key lessons learned from almost two decades of Aboriginal HIV and AIDS research. We explore opportunities and challenges, our experiences balancing our university-based "western" academic training with Indigenous, community-informed research, and, finally, the difficult and thorny question raised by Aveling (2013): "Should non-Indigenous researchers attempt to research with/in Indigenous communities or not" (p. 209)? Our chapter adds to this debate by examining community-based research and partnerships from the perspective of two insiders who work in the field. The lessons we have learned from the literature and our research experience may be of value to other diverse populations and to scholars engaging in research of local relevance.

Background

CAAN was incorporated in 1997. As a national nonprofit, nongovernmental body, CAAN's vision is "a Canada where First Nations, Inuit and Métis Peoples, families and communities achieve and maintain strong, healthy and fulfilling lives and significantly reduce HIV and AIDS, HCV, STBBIs, TB, Mental Health and related co-morbidity issues [and] where Aboriginal cultures, traditions, values and Indigenous knowledge are vibrant, alive, respected, valued and integrated into day-to-day life" (see www.caan.ca/about/). As authors of this chapter, and as a First Nation man and woman working with CAAN, it is culturally important for us to socially locate and introduce ourselves. Randy Jackson culturally identifies as *Anishinaabae* from the community of Kettle and Stony Point in southwestern Ontario, Canada. Renée Masching has Iroquois and Irish blood lines and identifies as an adoptee that was raised in a home with a first-generation Eastern European father and an English/Scottish-Canadian mother. We have worked together for more than 20 years and have collaborated closely on research initiatives led by CAAN. During this time, we have held roles as community stakeholders, knowledge users, research participants, staff, advisors, and research partners. We are currently research investigators on a number of different community-based research projects that involve working with Aboriginal and Indigenous people of diverse cultures, investigating equally diverse research topics.

In the research we design and conduct, we believe it is essential to bring attention to cross-cultural collaboration. Our communities inspire and challenge us to understand cultural diversity in dynamic ways, including, for example, ethnicity, gender diversity, age, class, sexual identity, HIV status, and physical ability. We know from this that it is extremely important to also recognize cultural differences with respect to the use of ceremony in research.[2] The diversity of worldviews across Indigenous cultures is vast and brings with it the ethical (and moral) imperative to "look . . . through the lens of Indigenous knowing and of the cultural forces that shaped the stories in the first place" (McLeod, 2007, p. 17; see also Brant Castellano, 2000). In this way, we recognize that "the term[s *Aboriginal* and] *Indigenous* may [themselves] be . . . homogenizing term[s], produced within colonization and [that may continue its] colonizing work by brushing over national or tribal differences" (Jones & Jenkins, 2008, p. 475; italics in original).

A Negative History of Research in the Aboriginal Community

As Indigenous community scholars working in the field, we are acutely aware of how the HIV-related research we have been involved with continues to unfold in the context of a negative history of research. The negative history of research exploitation in Aboriginal communities and the resulting harm it has caused is largely the result of, for example, culturally inappropriate and poorly informed data interpretation and meaning-making processes. In such cases, research was "conducted for or on local people rather than with them" (Blodgett et al., 2011, p. 265). Research data were often interpreted without the benefit of an insider's knowledge of community and cultural norms, mores, and processes. In fact, data analysis and interpretation were often guided by the cultural worldviews of the researcher(s) whose knowledge base was often informed by dominant Euro-Western values and norms. The high value placed upon remaining "objective," for example, was founded upon the bias that the worldview of the researcher was the norm by which others would be measured. Perhaps W. E. B. Du Bois (1903), an early 1900s African-American scholar, said it best when he wrote, "It is a peculiar sensation . . . this sense of always looking at one's self through the eyes of others, of measuring one's soul by the tape of a world that looks on in amused contempt and pity" (p. 2).

The history of negative research on Aboriginal peoples informed, for example, the design of the residential school system. In that instance researchers measured Aboriginal intelligence by culturally inaccessible teaching methods, labelled the communal responsibility to raise a child as neglect, and contributed to the stereotyping of Aboriginal peoples in Canada as incapable of caring for themselves. This was done without contextualizing the colonial impacts of loss of land, restricted hunting and destruction of traditional foodways, or the disrupted family and community relationships through the forced removal of children. Within this context, non-Aboriginal researchers built successful careers as "experts" on specific Nations with little or no direct engagement with the Aboriginal peoples who were their "research subjects." In fact, in many ways, the colonial intrusion experienced by Aboriginal peoples through research *on* (rather than *with*) has contributed to the disruption of traditional and cultural ways that continue to reverberate today. Not surprisingly, even today, some Aboriginal peoples continue to be reluctant to be involved in research.

For HIV-related research, these experiences are quickly changing, and Aboriginal peoples in Canada welcome research that draws on community-based approaches. More positive changes occurring as a result of community-based research approaches include more Aboriginal scholars leading research, the definition of rigorous research is evolving to include Indigenous epistemologies or ways of knowing; and Aboriginal communities are beginning to hold researchers accountable for their actions and, when necessary, issuing public statements challenging the Western-defined validity of analyses. As an approach, community-based research ensures that research is no longer in the exclusive domain of the academy. Community-based research offers not only a different way forward, but also one that is grounded in equitable and meaningful involvement of Aboriginal peoples in research.

Aboriginal communities have also made efforts to regulate research in their local jurisdictions as a means to protect their community from future negative research experiences (Brugge & Missaghian, 2006). Taking up this challenge, CAAN, like other national and international Indigenous community-based organizations, is committed to the development of models of culturally competent and sensitive research approaches (Burnette et al., 2011; Patterson, Jackson, & Edwards, 2006). Looking to the future, a strong desire for strengths-based rather than deficit-based inquiry is contributing a new dimension to our research.

Our approach has shifted from describing the social context of challenges faced by Aboriginal peoples in the context of HIV to exploring what positive factors or processes influence health. We are increasingly focused on concepts such as resiliency and the use of cultural mores as protective factors. We are also increasingly interested in how communities can positively address a range of social determinants of health, such as housing. This new orientation is guiding our current work, which is focused on exploring and investigating a range of wise practices (i.e., interventions) that best support and nurture Indigenous identity in health care and health services contexts. We value and use a social justice lens in our research. This moves CAAN away from investigating the social problems that contribute to HIV and AIDS in Aboriginal communities in Canada and toward identifying and seeking out solutions that are more congruent with our cultural perspectives, values, and worldviews.

Community-based Research with Aboriginal Communities

The promises of community-based research are expansive but are problematic when also working, as we do, with decolonizing and Indigenous methodologies. Although innovative when first introduced as a research approach, community-based research places enormous value and directs effort to successful community/academic collaborations. When conducting research *with* Aboriginal communities, the use of decolonizing and Indigenous methodologies raise important questions, including who speaks for Indigenous communities, who has the right to create Indigenous knowledge, how to respectfully include Indigenous community and cultural mores, the use of ceremony in research, and the role of cross-cultural collaboration in research.

Community-based research is defined in the literature as "a partnership approach to research that equitably involves community members, practitioners, and academic researchers in all aspects of the process, enabling all partners to contribute their expertise and share responsibility and ownership. Its purpose is to enhance understanding of a given phenomenon and to integrate knowledge gained with actions to improve health in the communities involved" (Israel et al., 2010, p. 2094). We know that community-based research is also congruent with Indigenous values because as a research approach, community-based research holds the potential to acknowledge, value, and enact different ways of honoring scientific, traditional, and cultural forms of knowing (Fletcher, 2003). It is widely regarded as a promising approach to produce relevant studies that inform program and policy design and action in Aboriginal communities in Canada (Cochran et al., 2008; Ritchie et al., 2013; Walters et al., 2009).

In this vein, community-based research values creating spaces and research structures that actively and meaningfully engage community insiders' perspectives in the formulation of the research questions and in developing and implementing research designs and processes (Blodgett et al., 2011). Several authors have suggested that a focus on the research *process* is as critically important as a focus on research outcomes (Cochran, et al., 2008; Edwards et al., 2008); indeed, these new research approaches are framed as an ethical obligation (Ball & Janyst, 2008; Dunbar & Scrimgeour, 2006). Certainly in the context of research *with* versus research *on* Aboriginal communities, it is the processes of building a collective understanding of the community(ies) of interest, the research topic, and the worldviews of the participants that will ensure the highest-quality outcomes.

Decolonizing and Indigenous Methodologies with Community-based Research

Indigenous peoples, since time immemorial, have always engaged in research. Knowledge of the world has been gathered, analyzed/interpreted, and passed on to others. Kincheloe and Steinberg (2008) describe Indigenous knowledges[3] as "a lived-world form of reason that informs and sustains people who make their homes in a local area" and who "construct ways of being and seeing in relation to their physical surroundings. Such knowledges involve insight into plant and animal life, cultural dynamics, and historical information used to provide acumen in dealing with the challenges of contemporary existence" (p. 136). Hart (2010) also notes Indigenous knowledges are holistic, dependent on relationships, connected to living and spiritual beings, honor many truths (individual, community, and nation), acknowledge that the land is sacred, and guide behavior in ways that respects that all things are equal.

The diversity of ways of knowing the world, through different sources and processes of learning, are reflected in the terminology of Indigenous knowledges. As often as knowledge may be written down, it is first and fore-most oral, conveyed in narrative and metaphorical language, and "validated through collective analysis and consensus building" (Brant Castellano, 2000, p. 26). In the context of research today, the term "Indigenous meth-odology" refers to research designs that are fully informed by community approaches to understanding the world. Indigenous ontologies (worldview) and epistemologies (ways of knowing) are actively reshaping the research approaches for working with Aboriginal communities in Canada. Data collection and analysis, for example, may include dreaming about the research, sharing data in ceremony to build understanding, oral interviewing with an emphasis on storytelling, and/or artistic expressions that are grounded in research designs. The survival of Indigenous communities and Indigenous peoples has been dependent upon adaptation—to land, environment—and these adjustments inform and guide Indigenous resistance to colonization. In this regard, methods that are used in "Western" research may also be adapted and used with Indigenous methodologies. It is the *why* and *how* these methods are used—how they are adapted—that potentially make the research design Indigenous and/or decolonizing.

However, Indigenous scholars have mixed optimism about efforts to "decolonize" research. Scholars have asked that if decolonizing is the end goal, then what exactly does that look like, and where does it lead? The idea of "decolonizing" is in itself complex and may in fact contribute as much to the essentialism of Indigenous or Aboriginal stereotypes as it is meant to push back against them. Calls to decolonize research are premised on the deficit-focused and negative research experiences of the past. As research-ers, often trained in North American/Western European-based academic institutions, there can be a tension between learning to be academically successful, requiring an understanding of the worldviews that under-pin academic research, and maintaining relationships and relating in the community. In this instance, the goal becomes seeking a balance between multiple worldviews and adapting the research designs to integrate both Indigenous knowledge and academic approaches.

It might be said that Indigenous researchers "walk in the worlds" of both academic and Indigenous knowledge (Tedlock, 2011). Jones and Jenkins (2008), writing of the divide between Indigenous and allied scholars, argue that this "[divide] is to be protected and asserted and is a positive site of productive methodological work" (p. 475). Walters and colleagues (2009) challenge community-based researchers to "retraditionalize" their research efforts. Wilson (2008) notes that although Indigenous scholars have extensively mapped the terrain of Indigenous ways of knowing, it is also equally important to apply this wisdom to inform different ways of collecting data and meaning-making to the research process. This raises the thorny question: Is the goal to work to reconcile the tensions across this difference (Cochran et al., 2008)? We ask whether resolving tensions are a necessary goal or whether efforts are a red herring to be cautiously approached.

Decolonizing and Indigenous methodologies "can be defined as research by and for Indigenous peoples, using techniques and methods drawn from the traditions and knowledge of those peoples" (Evans, Hole, Berg, Hutchinson, & Sookraj, 2009, p. 894). These methodologies both express an active commitment on the part of researchers to "acts of reclaiming, reformulating, and reconstituting Indigenous cultures and languages . . . to the struggle to become self-determining" (Smith, 1999, p. 142). The goal of research is to inspire social change for the benefit of Indigenous communities. Decolonizing and Indigenous methodologies are grounded in localized contexts, strive to increase Indigenous community participation in research, seek to disrupt colonial approaches to research, and work to create space for Indigenous voice (Kendall et al., 2011; Koster, Baccar, & Lemelin, 2012; Sherwood & Edwards, 2006). In this way, decolonizing and Indigenous approaches to research share values and a commitment to process that are congruent with community-based research approaches. All of these methodologies are value based and expansive with grounding in local contexts as their foundations. They are methodological orientations to research that are premised on collectivist or relational perspectives (Crofoot Graham, 2002).

Community-based Research Partnerships

As noted earlier, the inclusion of community-based research alongside decolonizing and Indigenous methodologies is not without its challenges. Nowhere do these tensions have more fruitful expression than through research grounded in Indigenous cross-cultural contexts. Efforts to decolonize and indigenize research also have implications for community/academic partnerships (Aveling, 2013; Cochran et al., 2008; Lincoln & Denzin, 2008) and pose challenges that may be familiar in the context of participatory research approaches. One of the most compelling questions being asked is whether non-Indigenous researchers should even attempt research with or in Indigenous communities (Aveling, 2013). Lincoln and Denzin (2008) also note that Indigenous peoples are asserting their rights to control research and that these stances likely "place serious restraints on Western scientists who wish to do work among them" (p. 564). In fact, many Indigenous communities are formally enacting control through, for example, the development of ethical guidelines and Indigenous ethics review (Brugge & Missaghian, 2006; Couzos et al., 2005; Patterson, Jackson, & Edwards, 2006). First Nation leadership in research set a national standard for Aboriginal research in the 1990s through the introduction of the OCAP™ Principles.[4] The principles of ownership, control, access and possession (OCAP™) from the conception to the completion of the research process informed the development of more inclusive Aboriginal research guidelines and also population-specific policies for Inuit, Métis, and local First Nations. Indigenous communities may additionally recommend that non-Indigenous researchers hand over or share their principal investigator status with community members who may or may not have academic credentials. Relinquishing leadership may have consequences for academic advancement (e.g., publication), yet community members may be better positioned to take up and use Indigenous forms of empiricism and other ways of knowing. A central element of a community-based research partnership also includes a commitment to capacity building (see chapter 7) that cultivates additional local cultural or research knowledge (Cochran et al., 2008).

The unpacking of these challenges compels Western researchers who wish to work with and in Indigenous communities to articulate research designs that implement non-exploitive research partnerships. This involves "[realizing] that it is not [a Western researcher's] place to conduct research within Indigenous contexts, but that [they] can use 'what [they] know'—rather than imagining what [they] know about Indigenous epistemologies or Indigenous experiences under colonization—to work as an ally with Indigenous researchers" (Aveling, 2013, p. 203). In other words, this strategy is focused on developing ways of relinquishing absolute Western control and making way for Indigenous researchers who bring knowledge and competency in Indigenous ways of knowing. Such approaches encapsulate the notion that the process by which researchers work collaboratively with and in Indigenous communities is as important, if not more important, than the actual knowledge that might be gained from implementing such a research design (Cochran et al., 2008).

Even this approach—the relinquishing of power to Indigenous research-ers—is problematic. Working across cultures, for example, can severely con-strain research partners who wish to work in Indigenous communities due to cultural mores and protocols that can limit sharing local knowledge with outsiders (Lincoln & Denzin, 2008). In this regard, as First Nation research-ers, the notion of insider/outsider applies: we are "insiders" as First Nations researchers; however, when working with other First Nations, Métis, or Inuit communities outside our own local communities, we are "outsiders." Such a perspective, when enacting decolonizing and Indigenous methodologies, is important and has implications in the context of community-based research.

Clearly, as others have already pointed out, there is a need for a different methodological approach for conducting research in and with Aboriginal communities (Kendall et al., 2011; Manson et al., 2004). Congruence between community-based research and Indigenous ways of knowing builds because it opens a collaborative research space (Strickland, 2006) rather than working to primarily resolve the tensions inherent in Indigenous cross-cultural collaboration. Further, we have found benefit in an approach that is structured to acknowledge diverse "interests and work toward one or more common goals while maintaining [our] own agendas" (Ansari, Phillips, & Zwi, 2002, p. 151). Green, Daniel, and Novick (2001) add to this concept by noting that successful partnerships are often premised on mutual trust that include openness, equality, and reciprocity; these values are lived rather than simply written into community/academic Principles for Research Collaboration (see Chapter 5) that guide the research project.

Although we too experience and recognize the complexity of these part-nerships, we assert that despite the tensions of collaboration, it is possible to conduct decolonizing research that draws on the strengths of Indigenous ways of knowing the world. The literature is rich with scholars who articu-late the benefits and the pressures of decolonizing research, and have been fruitfully mapping various strategies to address cross-cultural tensions in collaborative research models. For example, community-engaged schol-ars have highlighted the importance of local review and decision-making (Manson et al., 2004). They too have explored each stage of the research process, offering advice to achieve long-term partnership capacity to conduct research (Baldwin, Johnson, & Benally, 2009). In the past two decades, there has been noteworthy development of research approaches that support community relevance, participation, capacity building, and Indigenous community benefit (Ball & Janyst, 2008). For us, however, our continuing question is whether the resolutions of these tensions are an appropriate goal. Granted, although resolution to some tensions is desirable, more often than not our community research experiences have helped us to develop strategies to live with the tension and to invest our energies in the areas of Indigenous methodological development. Wilson (2008) has also challenged us to adopt this approach to research.

We see these tensions framed primarily by two complementary assertions. On the one hand, Indigenous peoples are rightfully concerned with whether their cultural knowledge, which is embedded in Indigenous methodologies, will be misappropriated. On the other hand, along with the objection to further research colonization, the level of cultural humility needed to achieve a meaningful understanding of cultural mores can be quite limiting. The literature attempts to address the issue of cross-cultural partnerships in several ways: by emphasizing the importance of Indigenous community relevance and benefit of research (Barnes, 2000); by exploring a range of applied strategies that support social transformation and the health and wellbeing of Indigenous communities (Blodgett et al., 2011); by working to empower Indigenous peoples as equal co-researchers (Braun et al., 2013); and by creating space in valuing Indigenous ways of knowing coupled with critical reflection and praxis (Browne, Smye, & Varcoe, 2005). In this vein, we highlight four research domain areas that are relevant to exploring cross-cultural research involving Indigenous peoples: (1) building effective research partnerships through reciprocal capacity building; (2) conceptualizing the research process with active and meaningful community involvement; (3) using the Medicine Wheel (an *Anishinaabae* symbol representing one's healing journey) as a symbol to both guide data collection and the development of understanding through analysis; and (4) developing meaningful and relevant dissemination tools that are accessible to community members.

Building Effective Research Partnerships through Mutual Capacity Building

Research capacity building is part of a larger strategy to address health in Aboriginal communities (Israel et al., 2010). Community-based research through community/academic partnerships are focused on co-learning (Blodgett et al., 2011; Braun et al., 2013). Entering into a community-based research partnership facilitates the opening of space for the meaningful inclusion of Indigenous approaches in research to blend these with Western research approaches. The intentional inclusion of learning opportunities for all team members to become both teachers and learners is critical to community-based research success. Alternately, having the opportunity to give and take is a humbling and confidence-building experience that can push team members outside of their "usual" roles. Further, another key strategy used by many outsider researchers is the practice of reflexivity (Getty, 2010). Such approaches open spaces for the meaningful inclusion of Indigenous approaches in research and the critical examination of the assumptions that underpin academic methodologies.

Aboriginal peoples in Canada and American Indians in the United States have begun to develop research engagement strategies (Manson et al., 2004; Brugge & Missaghian, 2006) and partnership or collaboration models based on values similar to the Principles of Research Collaboration described in chapter 5. Jacklin and Kinoshameg (2008) outline eight principles to advance the idea of successful, ethical partnerships with Aboriginal communities, including value of the partnership, empowerment strategies, community control, mutual benefit, wholism (the idea of "all my relations" in ways that embody Indigenous knowledges as collective, intergenerational, connected, and relational), action, communication, and respect. We must understand the value and necessity of strategies for developing and maintaining trust within the team and between communities.

Writing this chapter has offered us the opportunity to reflect across the research projects we have been involved in over the years and to consider how partnerships and capacity building has evolved. We continue to search for effective ways of solidifying community/university partnerships. Without attention to things such as trust building and reciprocal capacity building (i.e., shared understanding and language), partnerships can easily unravel. We invite and partner with allies—those colleagues who are non-Aboriginal and have demonstrated their willingness to contribute their knowledge—to learn with us and to develop ways of living with the tensions that arise in cross-cultural research. We also partner strategically with people who may have knowledge or experience that will assist us in achieving our research goals, but who may not be able or willing to work with Indigenous or decolonizing methodologies. Our strategic partners are often collaborators or co-investigators on our teams.

In our early projects, while developing our internal research capacity, we relied upon established academic researchers to partner with us and share leadership (see "The Influence of Stigma on Access to Health Services by Persons with HIV Illness" and "The Diagnosis and Care of HIV Infection in Canadian Aboriginal Youth" described earlier). In these two projects, CAAN led the participant recruitment process and contributed to—but did not lead—the analysis and knowledge dissemination. This helped to build on our experience and strong national networks. Partnerships continued to evolve with research project funds dispersed through universities to CAAN. Once our organization held these funds, we began to build our capacity to manage research funds, to hire research staff, and to engage community representatives in the development of research tools. With successive and successful projects, the development of grant proposals shifted to researchers positioned in CAAN, with allied academic partners sharing in the writing. Changes in funder policies made room for research leadership and administration to be fully in the hands of nonacademic institutions such as CAAN. This shifted the partnership dynamic again as CAAN became accountable for final decisions related to a research project.

As CAAN's internal capacity for academic research increased, so did our attention to the dynamics of community-based research and the need to engage in academic research with Aboriginal communities and community organizations. Early in the process we identified the need to ensure that university ethics review boards were balanced with our own internal process to offer advice from a committee of knowledgeable people who understood both university and community protocols. As we learned more about the research process as a whole, we also learned more about the points of (dis) connection between our community and academic worlds. We designed programs to engage our membership in community-based research through small projects and checked in with all team members during group meetings and individually to identify areas of confusion and/or tension. While we may have tried to resolve the tensions in our early projects, most often deferring to academic guidelines, ultimately we learned that too much was compromised in the pursuit of what would often be little more than superficial consensus.

One of CAAN's core research activities, through the "Aboriginal HIV and AIDS Community-Based Research Collaborative Centre (AHA Centre)," now focuses exclusively on reciprocal capacity building. We engage community to learn about academic protocols, proposal development, and research designs while at the same time engaging with our academic partners to learn about Indigenous and decolonizing methodologies, share in ceremony, and seek out opportunities to participate in community events. We also host a conference every other year to engage all of "our" research networks and invite the sharing of "Wise Practices in Aboriginal HIV and AIDS" community-based research. The goal in all of these activities is to (re)create safe spaces to share knowledge, to ask questions, and to build capacity to work with each other while respecting the others' perspectives.

Conceptualizing the Research Process

Research in Indigenous contexts requires the development of different ways of conducting research that are congruent with Indigenous worldviews (Walters et al., 2009; Wilson, 2008). Using First Voice methodologies (Aveling, 2013), conceptualizing research as ceremony (Wilson, 2008), incorporating "ecospiritual" perspectives (Coates & Gray, 2006), and research justice through sacred methodologies (Jolivette, 2015) are some examples of ways Indigenous scholars are responding to the critical need to reflect on research and the development of knowledge as a sacred practice. Drawing on the cultural assets of Indigenous communities, such as the use of elders and/or integration of appropriate ceremony into the research design (e.g., focus groups re-envisioned as sharing circles), potentially builds community understanding and shares control with them as the research process unfolds. The community/academic research team members who become involved with a research team need to know their community as a whole and specifically in the context the research is designed to investigate. In this regard, community-based research and Indigenous and decolonizing methodologies directly share common ground. Discussing how and why to use approaches in the research design so that team members can build consensus regarding the cultural processes is integral to success. During a project to explore cultural understanding of home, for example, we gathered digital stories from participants in four locations across Canada. In each of the project sites, we hired and trained peer research associates to work with our research team. Peer research associates were tasked, in part, to work with local elders to ground digital storytelling workshops with local ceremony and to contribute local cultural knowledge to aid in analysis and interpretation (e.g., analysis of data from each site was first completed by local team members who shared cultural ties with the participants and then brought that understanding of the local cultural and community context to guide interpretation of digital stories).

CAAN's research program is informed primarily by our membership. We hold an Annual General Meeting each year to report on our work and seek direction for future projects. Through this process we identify community leaders interested in specific research topics and the topics of most interest for further research. To meaningfully conceptualize our research, our first efforts focus on understanding why research on a topic is needed. We ask community leaders what they would like to know or understand more fully, and what particular issues or concerns are occurring in people's lives that might be related to the topic. We also ask: Is there an outcome that community members are hoping to see from the research?

We have used many approaches to develop research teams. We call upon, for example, community leaders who work with Aboriginal AIDS organizations based upon their areas of expertise, geographic location, and membership base. We also seek out individual community members who are living with HIV or AIDS and/or have lived experience related to the research topic. We seek out academic team members who we trust as allies, or who we believe could be potential allies, and who we would like to strategically partner with to best address the research topic. We have sent out recruitment posters for team members, held sharing circles to discuss a project idea and find out what others think about the topic, held retreats, and met in person and on the phone. These approaches continue to evolve throughout the research process and are driven by the needs of the project.

As we noted previously, the process is as important as the research outcomes, and is sometimes more important. What we mean by this is that the research is as much about how we engage, the processes we build into a research project for team communications, and how we maintain trust and share ideas. Methodological processes can be articulated, challenged, and refined most effectively when team members are comfortable working together. This is why meaningful engagement requires significant attention to each of the research team members' experience, knowledge, and history. We engage with team members by sharing articles about different research approaches and offering a small description of a methodology rather than simply the name of the approach, assuming that everyone will be interested in the development of the research design but not expecting everyone to speak out or respond to a draft of a proposal or publication. Finally, consistently creating space for decision-making input has also contributed to the effectiveness of our research. This approach has been used for most of the research projects in which we have been involved, but it comes at a cost in terms of time, labor, and additional resources. We work from an Indigenous perspective that values face-to-face partnership interaction, and therefore our research travel costs are often higher.

"Indigenizing" Data Collection and Analysis

Walters and colleagues (2009) call on those involved in Aboriginal community-based research to retraditionalize the research process. According to these authors, this "involves incorporating traditional and ancestral knowledge and methods into the formulation of research questions and the process of scientific inquiry" (p. 157). It is a position that has also found support in Jolivette's (2015) sacred methodologies and in Shawn Wilson's *Research Is Ceremony* (2008). Wilson (2008) effectively argues the need for data gathering and the development of analytic approaches that are congruent with Indigenous worldviews. These ways of conducting research are meant to support the maintenance of Indigenous identity in research contexts, to center and use Indigenous worldviews, and to be collaborative and anticolonial. However, one of the continuing challenges faced by Indigenous community/academic research teams is grounding such approaches in the literature. Though Indigenous scholars have produced an impressive body of knowledge that maps Indigenous consciousness, there is currently a dearth of literature that offers research teams direction specific to the development and use of methods and analytic processes that are anchored by Indigenous ways of knowing and meaning-making.

A far more common approach calls on researchers to indigenize their research processes by adapting existing Western methods using Indigenous knowledge. Tedlock (2011), who is herself Indigenous, reminds us that we "should walk in balance along the edges of these worlds. There is beauty and strength in being both: a double calling, a double love" (p. 337). It is an approach that is also consistent with principles of two-eyed seeing (Hatcher & Bartlett, 2010; Iwama et al., 2009). In other words, we draw on the strengths of Western ways of researching while actively and equitably blending these with Indigenous knowledge and ways of knowing the world. Several community/academic projects we are aware of have already successfully adapted Western methods and analysis to Indigenous contexts and include, for example, survey research approaches exploring cervical health among Native American women (Smith, Christopher, & McCormick, 2004), indigenizing narrative inquiry and storytelling approaches (Christensen, 2012; Jackson et al., 2014; Tedlock, 2011), and a range of arts-based methodological approaches to research (Blodgett et al., 2011).

One project we worked on incorporated both approaches (i.e., adapting methods and developing Indigenous analytic procedures) to explore resiliency among "two-spirit men" (a third gender that exists in many Aboriginal communities in Canada to describe individuals who self-identify as possessing both male and female attributes) in Ontario living long-term with HIV (Brennan et al., 2015). Despite the perception that two-spirit men test later, are sick more often, and die sooner than non-Aboriginal HIV-positive people in Canada, our community partners wanted to better understand the skills, resources, knowledge, and practices that were contributing to two-spirit men's health and wellbeing while living long-term with HIV. Exploring this question, our project adapted focus group methodology to sharing circles and used the *Anishinaabae* symbol of the Medicine Wheel—because it represents one' healing journey—to stimulate dialogue and conversation about strengths, assets, and resiliency. We also used the Medicine Wheel later in the project to develop a research analysis process to ground our emerging understanding of what it meant to live resiliently with HIV on a long-term basis. Our analytic process involved several stages: (1) we offered team members cross-cultural training on the teachings of the Medicine Wheel; (2) we developed a codebook in which, line-by-line, all data expressing similar patterns were coded using NVivo 10.0; (3) we used principles of participatory analysis (Flicker & Nixon, 2014; Jackson, 2008) to select key quotes under each code and map these to the Medicine Wheel in areas that expressed similar meaning (i.e., statements about resiliency that focused on physical, emotional, mental, and spiritual aspects of self); and (4) we grouped codes that represented a relationship to other codes and labelled them according to the teachings of the Medicine Wheel (e.g., statements about the importance of Aboriginal identity or worldview). These relationships were meant to express the constellation of their component code parts and their relationship to our study question. We found that by using the cultural symbols of the Medicine Wheel we provided a more attuned and structured way to interpret and understand data in ways that foregrounded Indigenous worldviews. In other words, the analytic process can potentially shift the way researchers come to understand, write, speak about, and present scholarly research focused on Aboriginal HIV resiliency through the worldviews of those most directly affected.

Despite our success using Indigenous knowledge in this project, we experienced challenges that required us to work as a team. Based on our experience, we have several suggestions that may be useful for researchers working with two-spirit communities: to work effectively, we needed to agree on working terminology (e.g., defining "two-spirit" for academics and community); we experienced differing conceptions of research ethics given the focus on Indigenous knowledge (e.g., foregrounding Indigenous worldviews as an ethical imperative); we worked across differences in terms of understanding Indigenous worldviews versus settler identity, particularly in relationship to traditional two-spirit knowledge; and we used techniques to enhance the reciprocal learning of both community providers and the research team. Here, the quality of our community–academic partnership helped to keep the project moving forward as we worked as a team to address the question of whether Indigenous knowledge is as equally valued and as valid as Western ways for developing knowledge. In other words, as a team we needed to actively work towards avoiding "intellectual arrogance . . . and paternalistic practices" (Aveling, 2013, pp. 203–204) that might have stymied our efforts.

"Indigenizing" Dissemination Strategies

Ideally, dissemination about a research project occurs throughout the life of a project because this is foundational to increasing the knowledge base and community capacity to take effective action aimed at social transformation. To accomplish this, the literature highlights effective knowledge-translation strategies to accommodate the urgent need for timely and appropriate research information. Drawing on the Indigenous Peoples' Health Research Centre's (IPHRC) report *Sharing What We Know about Living a Good Life: Indigenous Knowledge and Knowledge Translation Summit* (Kaplan-Myrth & Smylie, 2006), approaches developed by CAAN (Masching, Allard, & Prentice, 2006), and those in the literature (Ball & Janyst, 2008), our work builds on and works with community, academic, and policy stakeholders to inform strategies primarily directed at three broad audiences: community, academic, and policy.

Our recent research experiences suggest to us that the use and value of cultural symbols or cultural approaches to sharing and transferring knowledge offers unique ways to write, speak about, and present findings in ways more congruent with Aboriginal worldviews. This potentially facilitates the goal of knowledge translation, exchange, and uptake of research findings in communities of interest. Along with the development of project reports, which are familiar formats for policy audiences, we have incorporated arts-based approaches such as videos with research participants or community research associates to share the research findings. Our project focus on resilience among two-spirit men, for example, used data visualization and information architecture to graphically present findings using a Medicine Wheel. An online web space was created for community members (as well as other audiences) to interactively explore our research findings in ways that made sense to them. Another project we are involved in will explore experiences and responses to depression among Aboriginal peoples living with HIV and AIDS. Here we plan to use storytelling, because stories and storytelling are conceptualized within Aboriginal communities as healing. They actively center Indigenous knowledges, and can also offer culturally congruent information about health challenges to participants and others (Jackson et al., 2014). Similarly, in another project we undertook a scoping review of global decolonizing and Indigenous methodological literature and drew on the aesthetic of oral storytelling and the power of documentary film to disseminate findings (Worthington et al., 2013). For this project, we hosted a research team-sharing circle, video-recorded our dialogue, and then selected key themes to share with wider audiences (visit CAAN's YouTube channel at www.youtube.com/user/CdnAboriginalAIDS).

In addition, as Aboriginal scholars, we are also interested in reaching academic audiences; our success as researchers is measured in part through publications. Given early difficulties with the publication process (e.g., lack of culturally attuned reviewers that could fairly assess Aboriginal community-based HIV research), we launched and continue to edit our own peer-reviewed and fully indexed journal (see the *Canadian Journal of Aboriginal Community-Based HIV/AIDS Research* at www.caan.ca/canadian-journal-of-aboriginal-based-hivaids-research/cjacbr-volume-1-2006/). For the journal, we invite publications that meet specific criteria (i.e., community-based research, Aboriginal, HIV-related) and administer the work of a blinded peer-review process whose committee membership is made up of academic and community members. In this context, our work maintains focus on capacity building, and the meaningful engagement of community throughout the research process, including data collection, analysis, and dissemination. We actively encourage authors to include community voices in their publications submitted to our journal. Community members have also begun to join in the process of writing academic journal articles in addition to contributing to community dissemination events. We also actively develop our own expertise to support community members to contribute to the publication process (Peltier et al., 2011).

Ways Forward

Early in the development of CAAN's (2006) research capacity, we wrote a paper titled "Researching Ourselves to Life." This was in some ways our manifesto and declaration that after being researched to death by "outside" others, we were embracing the potential of research to restore ourselves. More than 15 years into our research program, we have witnessed the evolution of membership support for research and have learned to develop research partnerships that support our vision of healthy, thriving Aboriginal communities. With respect to cross-cultural collaboration in community-based research, and despite continuing challenges, we firmly believe that there is more common ground than tension. As we reflect on the promise and challenge of community-based research in Indigenous contexts, we offer two useful approaches to move forward.

First, we need to continue to find and develop more effective ways of solidifying community/academic partnerships. If there is not a focus on building trust and reciprocal capacity (i.e., shared cultural understanding and language), partnership can very easily unravel. We need to devise ways of *living with* rather than *resolving* these tensions. We are concerned that the erasure of differences across multiple ways of knowing might reflect a colonizing approach. Rather than adopting and holding all knowledge as valued and equal, we wish instead to create a level playing field where all knowledges are valued for their contribution.

Second, we must continue to develop and weave Indigenous knowledge throughout the entire research process. This approach recognizes the fundamental nature of knowledge and its development as a sacred endeavor. As we work toward embedding ceremony in our research processes, we must also be cognizant of the challenges this poses as we work cross-culturally. That is, we must be sensitive to the discomfort that this causes for those "outside" a particular culture. For us, community-based research allows us to find ways forward that are meaningful and ethical and that advance social justice.

Section IV
Future Challenges

9. Enacting Social Justice

In this chapter we highlight the importance of enacting social justice in community-based research. We explore the roles of key stakeholders in academia, the community, and community organizations in pursuing social justice agendas. At the same time, we raise questions about the challenges to and possibilities for democratic leadership and issues of oppression. We contemplate the question: Is community-based research research for social justice, or is it socially just research? We end this chapter with a focus on change. In 2005 Norman Denzin and Yvonna Lincoln, who are well known for their contributions to the theory of qualitative research, described the stages of development of qualitative research in the social sciences and humanities. They saw 2005 as a time that reflected "critical conversations about democracy, race, gender, class, nation-states, globalization, freedom and community" (Denzin & Lincoln, 2005, p. 3). Increasingly since that time, researchers and communities have engaged in these critical conversations. While community-based research reflects an interest in democracy, oppression, and change, we are mindful that community-based research cannot become the new orthodoxy in the field of research, nor do we want it to become an instrument for enacting social justice.

Essentials of Community-based Research by Vera Caine and Judy Mill, 109–120. © 2016 Left Coast Press, Inc. All rights reserved.

Key Stakeholders and Gatekeepers in the Community and Academy

For Francisco Ibáñez-Carrasco (2004), community-based research "is science at the service of community interests" (p. 49). While we agree with this perspective, we also wonder about framing research as a service, which entails an act of servitude that may not fully acknowledge the multiple ways in which community-based research is initiated and conducted or the impact that it can have on those involved in the field. We have been involved in projects that primarily served the interests of the community, but we also have initiated projects that had conflicting and competing interests within the community. We are mindful that neither the community nor academics have the sole responsibility or ability to identify, define, and dismiss issues. For us it is key that community-based research is understood and realized within a community and that the diversity, dissent, and also resistance to projects are acknowledged. Community members, organizations, and researchers might bring very different understandings, not only of the identified issues but also in their conceptualization of justice and equity. Often these differences represent diverse vantage points and are not necessarily in conflict, yet at other times they are. Understanding and considering these various values and the validity of the issues is important and an inevitable challenge and tension when one is engaging in community-based research (Walton et al., 2014).

Without clearly understanding differences in values and conceptualizations of issues, it is difficult to distinguish clear roles and responsibilities for those involved in community-based research. Researchers need to address fundamental questions about what community means, how to define community, and the relationship between community and research. While this is particularly important when researchers are strangers to the community, it is equally important for those who belong to the community to identify their inherent values. Intentionally and unintentionally, researchers and community members are influenced by their values, as well as their history and social position in relation to the community and the existing dynamics within the community. These dynamics can shape a few basic questions: Who should participate in the research? How should those selected participate? What are people's specific contributions? These dynamics can shape the roles of those involved at all stages of the partnership, including the engagement, formalization, mobilization, and maintenance of partnerships (Cargo & Mercer, 2008).

Throughout our work, we have learned how important it is to focus on the collaborative aspects of community-based research. For example, in the project we recently completed (Mill et al., 2014a) to explore the clinical mentorship of nurses as an intervention in HIV care, it was important to understand the local reality of nurses' workloads and the political and social support they received for participation in the project. It was also important to consider the reasons why communities refused or requested their participation within the project. In one Canadian jurisdiction we were unable to engage in capacity building with registered nurses despite their interest. It became evident over time that senior personnel representing the health authority did not feel that HIV care was a priority and did not share our belief that nurses should be able to choose between different continuous educational opportunities in their area of practice. Even though we had strong partnerships with AIDS service organizations and people living with HIV in these areas, we were unable to overcome this challenge in some jurisdictions. We learned a great deal from this project in terms of access to continuing education, the importance of HIV care, and the bureaucratic nature of decision-making in which decisions are often made by those far removed from clinical practice sites. We also learned a lot about collaboration, values, and power.

In hindsight, there are things we could have done differently. In future projects we will try to develop collaborations with stakeholders who might not share our values or see the importance of issues that others in the community have identified. Strand, Marullo, Cutforth, Stoecker, and Donohue (2003) identify seven useful tasks or functions of collaboration:

1. Mobilizing resources
2. Building multiplex (deep) relationships among collaborators
3. Creating appropriate divisions of labor
4. Managing information and authority relations (this is so important!)
5. Devising rules and control mechanisms for undertaking research projects
6. Managing external relationships
7. Constructing sustainable mechanisms

Building on these seven tasks, we must also involve multiple community members in actual research activities (including publishing), to develop jointly agreed-upon research principles (see chapter 5), to engage in training opportunities, and to create diverse research teams with skill sets in collaboration.

For Terry Trussler and Rick Marchand (2005), who work with the community-based research center for gay men's health in Vancouver, Canada, "[t]he question of whether or not CBR [community-based research] studies should be considered contributions to formal knowledge hardly matters when such collaborations clearly contribute to improvements in practice . . . . The process is as important as the outcome" (pp. 52–53). Though it is critical to acknowledge the importance of the process, funding agencies and those involved in community-based research often want clear outcomes, or at a minimum useful results. In addition, funding agencies often do not grant sufficient funds for research team members to write about the research process after the outcomes and results are disseminated.

Beyond considering processes, it is vital to acknowledge that particular roles within research projects also reflect different degrees of power and control. Everyone involved needs to recognize and acknowledge these power differentials; at a minimum, there needs to be an explicit acknowledgment of these differences. At best, project roles and their associated power can be negotiated to offset existing power differentials. Wolf (1996) outlines three perspectives on power that reflect one's positionality as outsider, insider-outsider, or outsider-within. These positionalities shape:

1. the extent of privileged identity (or identities) within societal social norms and within the specific community and academic relationship;
2. the research process itself: who defines the research design, decision making processes, and levels of power sharing; and
3. the representation and writing of the findings: whose voices are privileged and being heard.

We also add to this that power shapes what counts as knowledge. At the same time, it is important to take risks, to improvise along the way, and to recognize that "[k]nowledge emerges only through invention and reinvention, through the restless, impatient, continuing, hopeful inquiry [people] pursue in the world, with the world, and with each other" (Freire, 1989, p. 58). Perhaps this is not unlike what Maxine Greene (1995) offers us when she reminds us that

in thinking of community, we need to emphasize the process words: making, creating, weaving, saying, and the like. Community cannot be produced simply through rational formulation nor through edict. Like freedom, it has to be achieved by persons offered the space in which to discover what they recognize together and appreciate in common; they have to find ways to make intersubjective sense. (p. 39)

In this way, collaboration is a way of being in community-based research that forefronts relationships and attends to processes.

Challenges to and Possibilities for Democratic Leadership

Community-based research builds on the traditions of participatory research (see chapter 1), which emerged from working with people who were oppressed in developing countries (Fals-Borda & Rahman, 1991; Hall, 1993) as well as the Brazilian educator and philosopher Paulo Freire's (1989) work on democracy and democratic citizenship. Since this early work, other scholars have linked democratizing practices with community-based work. For example, Patti Lather (2013) writes:

method is political and that is a good thing to think with as we explore how much the development of a counter science "on our own terms" can be community based, community sustaining, and community serving in ways that might help alter the structures of institutions in more expansive democratizing ways. (p. 642)

It is important to understand that we are most interested in the spirit of democracy (Paszek, 2012). Thus, democracy is not the end goal or outcome of the work we do; instead, democracy is, as pragmatist and well-known educational thinker John Dewey (1916) points out, always in progress. This too means that we need to remain attentive to the ongoing practices of community-based research in which the responsibility for each project is shared.

While the responsibilities for achieving a shared sense of democracy is significant, researchers and community members must inquire into their own experiences and understandings of privilege. There also is a need to be aware of how privilege shapes the ongoing and long-term commitment to research projects and communities (Chavez et al., 2008). Patti Lather (1986), feminist and postmodernist, talks about reciprocal reflexivity and critique, arguing that both activities "guard against the central dangers of praxis oriented empirical work: imposition and reification on the part of the researcher" (p. 265). In addition, reflexivity can guard against the imposition and reification on the part of the communities or community members. For Paulo Freire (1989), it was important that authentic thinking occurred through communication and engagement, while feminist researchers show us that it also is about the intentional involvement of participants or communities in the interpretation of meaning or in the reflection on experiences.

It is critical to think about democratic practices in relation to community-based research, and therefore it is important to follow Biesta's (2011) argument that

> [t]here is a need to shift the focus of research, policy and practice from the teaching of citizenship towards the different ways in which young people "learn democracy" through their participation in the contexts and practices that make up their everyday lives, in school, college and university, and in society at large. (p. 6)

This is significant because Biesta links democracy to everyday practices as well as citizenship, which is not just the legal status of people within a state, but also develops through the opportunity to significantly shape life within a community or society (Simon, 2001). In Dewey's (1916) classic text *Democracy and Education*, he advocates that citizens actively engage in seeking communal solutions for shared issues. Dewey was well aware that this was not an easy task in face of the diversity of backgrounds and interests within communities. Giroux (2003) links "hope, democracy, education and the demands of a more fully realized democracy" (p. 42); for him, a new theoretical language of social action is necessary.

We cannot underestimate the importance of democratic practices, but these practices also need to be reciprocal (Sernak, 2009). We are reminded of British sociologist and feminist Ann Oakley's words that there is "no intimacy without reciprocity" (1981, p. 49). It is our experience that ethics boards at times struggle with notions of reciprocity and intimacy, raising questions about boundary issues and potential therapy. This is particularly challenging for us; we see community-based research as a long-term commitment to communities, whereby participants and those involved in research become friends and close colleagues, or work with us as graduate students. Who we are within projects is also influenced by our own life narratives. For Maxine Greene (1995), "it is on that primordial ground that we recognize each other, that ground on which we are in direct touch with things and not separated from them by the conceptual lenses of constructs and theories" (p. 75).

Linking reciprocity and intimacy to democracy also means that we pay close attention to people and live in ways that reflect relational ethics (Bergum & Dossetor, 2005) and care (Bateson, 1995). In this way we acknowledge not only our personal bonds, but also mutual responsibilities to care and respond in deeper ways to the everyday issues faced by and within communities; these are opportunities to show that we care for others.

> Democracy, we realize, means a community that is always in the making. Marked by an emerging solidarity, a sharing of certain beliefs, and a dialogue about others, it must remain open to newcomers, that too long have been thrust aside. (Greene, 1995, p. 39)

Challenging Oppression

It is impossible to talk about community-based research without acknowledging existing and potential oppression. We see oppression as the unjust use of power or authority, which can deeply shape the lives of people and communities. Practitioners in community-based research are aware that

> oppressive structures can be reproduced within research, particularly the potential for the reproduction of gender, racial/ethnic and socioeconomic inequalities and power differentials. . . . Academic researchers represent centers of power, privilege, and status within their formal institutions, as well as within the production of scientific knowledge itself. Researchers also may have power and privilege from their class, education, racial/ethnic backgrounds, or other identity positions. Both of these positionalities (power and privilege) have the potential for reproducing systemic health inequities and disadvantaging community partners. (Muhammad et al., 2014, p. 2)

These disadvantages may represent oppressive conditions if they are not addressed, or if researchers and community members are not intentionally awake to them.

Only more recently have others begun to write about these complexities within their research and the populations they work with. In 2008,

Cargo and Mercer carried out a critical review of the exiting literature and found that though community-based research reports were able to build capacities, they did not link this ability to a framework of empowerment and ownership. For McLaren (1989), who draws on Foucault's work, it is important to understand that truth is always constructed in relationships with others, and that it is negotiated. McLaren argues "that praxis (informed actions) must be guided by phronesis (the disposition to act truly and rightly). This means, in critical terms, that actions and knowledge must be directed at eliminating pain, oppression and inequality, and at promoting justice and freedom" (p. 182). Embedded in this understanding is that community-based research links to critical education.

Community-based research is also about co-learning, attending to issues of social inequities, and also about empowerment (Israel et al., 1998). Vera has often thought about the history and processes that mark the Délı̨nę Uranium Research project. This research clearly was a response to social justice matters and the mounting questions within the community about the actual and potential future impact of uranium and radium exposure on people, animals, and the land. Community members realized that few people outside of their community knew about this part of Canadian history and how Canada was implicated in the bombing of Hiroshima. As part of the project, community members developed a book titled *If We Had Only Known . . .* (Délı̨nę First Nations, 2005a), which reflected the oral history project and told the stories of individual families who had lived and worked as ore carriers along the transportation route. In this way the experiences within the community of Délı̨nę were no longer silenced, and the stories played a significant part in reimaging a different history. For Drevdahl (2002),

> [c]ommunity can be a source of strategies for hindering, but, more important, for changing oppressive conditions. Thus, community becomes a location where one stays because it replenishes one's ability to endure and resist, it is a place where one can envision alternative worlds and ways of being. (p. 16)

It was this imaginative capacity to tell a different story that affected the project in Délı̨nę.

Community-based research holds the potential for people to illuminate the complexity of issues they experience, as well as to address issues that have been neglected. For Denzin (1999), community-based research can decenter academic authority, while for Mayan and Daum (2014), this approach is change oriented and challenges the *us and them* dichotomy that continues to shape much of research. However, this potential can be undermined if those involved in community-based research do not acknowledge the power related to the positionality of researchers: power that reflects complex intersections of gender, sexual orientation, ability, culture, racial/ethnic, educational, and other forms of identity.

Research for Social Justice, or Socially Just Research?

Although community-based research seeks social justice and has emancipatory purposes (Mayan & Daum, 2014), we also must ask whether it is socially just research. This means that our research can be guided by shared ownership, and that social problems or issues are analyzed in collaboration with the community. Unintentionally, this can be very problematic. Vera recalls her very first community-based research project that was part of her master's work, when she explored the experiences of Aboriginal women living with HIV. One of the community agencies providing services to people living with HIV referred a participant to Vera. Several months later, the agency requested a copy of the raw data and felt that they had ownership in the project. This posed a significant challenge to Vera, who felt that her first responsibility was to her research participants. At the same time, Vera was well aware that the findings of her work had greater potential to influence the social determinants of health if she worked closely with the agency. After conversations with the participants, Vera decided not to share any of the tape-recorded conversations or information but instead ensured that the agency had access to the final thesis and any publications. As a result of this dialogue, some of the research participants engaged more fully with the agency without disclosing that they were research participants. For Vera this interaction highlighted the complex understanding of ethics and commitments in socially just research.

In the last few years the boundaries between researcher and research, academic and activist, have become blurry (Banks et al., 2013). At times this blurriness has caused tensions; at other times, it has raised questions of loyalty. Perhaps issues of betrayal are at play in these instances. Patti Lather (1986) argues that "searching for an emancipatory approach to research ... [and] what it means to do empirical research in an unjust world" (p. 257) looks more closely at critical or praxis-oriented research. For her, praxis means "the dialectical tension, the interactive, reciprocal shaping of theory and practice which I see at the center of an emancipatory social science" (p. 258). While for Lather this involves connecting research methodology to theoretical concerns and commitments, praxis is a useful way to think in community-based research. Praxis can be understood as the dialectical relationship between theoretical understandings and community experiences that both aim to initiate and sustain social change. When we engage in this way, the aim of our engagement is not an innocent practice, but a political one. Drawing on other scholars, Sarah Flicker and colleagues (2008a) recognize that, "[community-based research] strives to marry the twin goals of community development with knowledge generation to achieve social justice ends" (p. 240).

It is important that researchers attend to both distributive justice and procedural justice (Minkler, 2010), as both are relevant to addressing disparities and inequities. This is strongly shaped by the complex relationship between power and evidence. Freudenberg and Tsui see this complex relationship reflected in the following questions about policy change:

1. What are the benefits and limits of the scale of community as a focus of policy change and when are other scales more appropriate venues for policy work?
2. Who are the appropriate participants in policy change initiatives? What are appropriate roles for various players in the policy change process? What are the procedures that allow meaningful participation by necessary constituencies?
3. What is the role of research (or scientific evidence) in policy change? In what circumstances does evidence drive policy change and when are other levers of change needed? (2014, p. 11)

Focus on Change

In community-based research the connection to policy or practice change is often critical, and is one of the key reasons community members engage. Yet there is no linear relationship between community-based research and change; rather, we see multiple tensions between evidence and change that are most often affected by politics and guided by values, morals, and many other interests. For this reason we must demonstrate long-term commitments to the communities we work with and become actively involved in the life of the community, regardless of funded research projects. For some, community-based research builds a natural infrastructure for influencing local policy (O'Brien & Whitaker, 2011).

David Berg, one of the community members we worked closely with, had very particular notions of power and change, notions that were attached to the need to act and behave in certain ways. For him, it was important that we maintained a presence in his life, that he was well aware of our every step, and that we trusted his instincts and accepted his informal leadership. His sustained commitment to the AIDS Service Organization, with which we worked closely, was important because David carried a long institutional memory of things that had been tried, of change that had been initiated and supported, and also change that had failed. While David did not hold a formal position within the organization, his understandings were important.

Understanding how community members and organizations interact is also important, particularly, as Wallerstein and Duran (2006) argue, because

> [p]olicy change, using the research data, at a community level may exactly depend on community-based organizations who can represent the community's vision, and who has the authority to take ownership of the problem and history of activism to make change happen. (p. 318)

While the vision and direction for change are critical goals in community-based research, participatory research in general aims at three types of changes: "1) development of a critical consciousness of both researcher and participants; 2) improvement of the lives of those involved in the research process; and 3) transformation of fundamental societal structures and relationships" (Heffner, Zandee, & Schwander, 2003, p. 129). What is not well established is how participatory or community-based research can act as a structural framework for change (Wallerstein & Duran, 2006). This is important, for community-based research can be what others have called a "local trap," which is a "tendency to assume that a particular scale—in this case, the community—is inherently more desirable than others, even if other (higher) levels are more influential determinants of health and are more effective starting points for policy change" (Freudenberg & Tsui, 2014, p. 12). Although this understanding should not minimize or dismiss community-based research, it is important to purposefully situate local communities historically, socially, culturally, and politically within a broader landscape (Cacari-Stone, Wallerstein, Garcia, & Minkler, 2014).

This way of situating communities is important because the issues that are the phenomena of research in community-based research do not necessarily reflect or become policy or political issues. Often it is up to those involved to convert the issues under investigation into political issues and to make policy recommendations (Gamble & Stone, 2006). At the same time,

> rather than asking whether policy has changed, a more fruitful question might be, "How did the [partnership's] work to *improve the policy environment* for this issue?" or "How successful was the [partnership] in *taking the necessary steps toward the policy change?*" (Minkler, 2010, p. S85; italics added)

As researchers, community members, and organizations engage in conversations about community-based research, it is inevitable that discussion about change happens. Within these discussions it is important to resist notions and pressures of conformity, instead ensuring that these discussions become "the practice of freedom, the means by which men and women deal critically and creatively with reality and discover how to participate in the transformation of their world" (Richard Shuall as cited in Freire, 1989, p. 15). Cargo and Mercer (2008) point out that increasing collaboration might be a vehicle to sustain and leverage greater commitment to using research findings to take action and ultimately to engage in change. Scarinci, Johnson, Hardy, Marron, and Partridge (2009) go as far as saying that "[i]f transformation does not occur, we, as researchers, failed. In most instances this failure is due to lack of equalizing power and true involvement of all parties in the process" (pp. 221–226). After engaging in community-based research, we feel we are just beginning to learn how to leverage change but also when to step back and situate our work in new ways, highlighting the complexity and messiness of socially just research and research for social justice. In our final chapter, we look ahead to areas that require ongoing work and commitment.

10. Ways Forward

Throughout this book we have provided several examples, challenges, and possibilities from our experiences with community-based research projects. Much of our work is situated in the field of HIV, as well as alongside communities who experience significant marginalization. We concur with Rhodes that

> HIV prevention research and practice have been at the forefront of community engagement and partnership and [community-based participatory research]. Early on in the HIV epidemic, gay men and their close allies mobilized to promote action and lead the way in sound approaches to community engagement in the design, implementation, evaluation, translation, and dissemination of prevention interventions. In fact, we now have a critical mass of current and recent HIV prevention intervention studies that have applied innovative approaches to engagement, partnership, and [community-based participatory research]. (2014, p. 7)

Looking across the field of community-based research we see that it is important not only to acknowledge and celebrate the depth of knowledge about processes that have been developed but also to identify what remains a work in progress.

In this chapter we attend to the "So what?" questions about community-based research that we know academics, students, community members and organizations, policymakers, and frontline practitioners will ask. We reflect upon the roots of community-based research and contemplate further the notion of praxis, and finally return to the criteria for judging community-based research. We also build on key issues in thinking about

Essentials of Community-based Research by Vera Caine and Judy Mill, 121–131. © 2016 Left Coast Press, Inc. All rights reserved.

and developing mutually agreed-upon research principles as one way to highlight the relational and collaborative work central in community-based research: work that aims not only to address social justice issues but also to engage in socially just research. We end this chapter with a reflection upon the promises of community-based research and ultimately ask questions about how this work can and does shift inequities and oppression.

Returning to the Roots of Community-based Research

Returning to the roots of community-based research entails reconsidering its epistemological, ontological, and ethical commitments. Yet it also means that we need to look again at the diverse understandings of community, research, and participation. Israel, Schulz, Parker, and Becker's (1998) definition of community-based research is widely accepted: "Community-based research . . . focuses on social, structural, and physical environmental inequities through active involvement of community members, organizational representatives, and researchers in all aspects of the research" (p. 173). The focus on inequities that can be identified and named is evident, as is the involvement of communities or their members in all phases of the research project. If we reconsider the principles on which community-based research is built, we also need to emphasize the long-term commitment to collaboration. Several researchers have pointed out how challenging this commitment can be, for communities are not homogenous, nor do they share the same values, understandings, or experiences; there are times when some of the differences are irreconcilable.

Yet, community members, organizations, and researchers must be willing to fulfill their commitments despite the tensions and challenges they encounter. If community-based research honors Paulo Freire's (1989) notions of critical consciousness or conscientization, then we also need to acknowledge that we as academics are part of relationships, contexts, and situations in which we may not know what is or might be happening. We will continue to find ourselves in places and spaces that can be unsettling and uncomfortable. In these moments it is important to engage and commit to critical dialogues and avoid oppressive and dehumanizing actions. Despite these challenges, when community-based research is done "with an attitude of humility and real respect for how much the community has to teach us, [community-based participator research] can indeed be an exhilarating path" (Stoecker, 2008, p. 118).

Researchers positioned within the academy continue to face very particular challenges when they engage in community-based research, some
of which have been described by Etmanski, Hall, and Sawson (2014):

1. The challenges of working from an academic location
2. Who are the learners? Who are the teachers? Who is the community?
3. Can we re-story the word *research*?
4. Respecting the diversity of knowledge cultures

Each one of these points alludes to very particular contexts and challenges
that must be continuously addressed. Vera recalls one of her recent conversations with representatives of a community organization. The community
organization contacted Vera and some of her colleagues because they were
interested in identifying and implementing an intervention for children
at risk for sexual exploitation. During the initial conversation, Vera realized that the community agency thought the researchers would have the
solutions for the problems they encountered. This was an uncomfortable
place for Vera, as she did not know the agency well. She did not know
the children, youth, families, and other agencies that intersected with the
children's lives. After several conversations, the community agency and
Vera negotiated a different approach to the agency's request for an intervention. Using this approach, Vera, along with colleagues from different
disciplinary backgrounds, the agency, the children, and their families, all
held relevant knowledge and experiences. Instead of imposing an intervention, the agency decided to engage in community-based research with a
focus on participatory action. In this way the community agency, but most
important the children and their families, were central to all aspects of the
work, including the development of a possible intervention.

As research alongside community agencies unfolds, Vera and Judy are
reminded how important it is to place communities before the academia.
Doing so helps to "de-romanticize the nearly bankrupt concept of community that is currently applied to almost any gathering of persons, ideas, and
products to add a patina of authenticity" (Joseph, 2002, as cited in Ibáñez-
Carrasco & Riano-Alcala, 2009, p. 73). This is also important because
many communities who have relied on expert advice (often outside of their
community) have realized that expert-driven research has "proven ineffec-
tive and communities across North America are demanding that they be
given great[er] decision-making power over studies that take place in their
midst" (Flicker et al., 2008c, p. 106). Placing communities in the center of

our work also shifts the focus away from problems and toward possibilities. In community-based research, the strengths of all stakeholders must be identified and diversity must be respected to address issues relevant to the community. This has, at times, been called a shift to "collaborative inquiry, co-operative research, or appreciative inquiry" (Edwards et al., 2008, p. 188); for us, it is a shift that honors the principles of community-based research.

Over the last few years, research has increasingly become commodified and considered a means to achieve a particular end or outcome. It is more difficult to locate funding for research driven by curiosity, research that is often messier and less predictable. This is particularly significant to community-based research that seeks to foster social justice, public participation, and democratic citizenship. We also see the demand by funding agencies to have clear knowledge mobilization or dissemination plans. For us, these plans are difficult to quantify at the beginning of a community-based research project when the findings of the proposed research are still unclear. We also find that priorities shift continuously within communities. A research priority identified when a funding application is submitted might no longer be the community's key priority when funding is received. The length of time it takes to obtain adequate funding is a deterrent for communities to invest large amounts of resources into the development of partnerships. The inability of communities to invest significant resources, such as time, is intensified when it is unclear whether the proposed research will be funded at all.

These challenges raise questions for us that are challenging to reconcile: How do we establish and maintain partnerships when no funding for a project has been received? Could shifting community priorities result in the abandonment of long-planned community-based research? What is our and the community's responsibilities in these moments? How do we determine key stakeholders in community-based research when long-term funding does not exist for many partners or organizations? In working with communities, we also see the frequent shift of staff to new positions and people moving out of the community. How are projects, ideas, and partnerships transitioned within communities, but also within the academy? Given this context, how do we ensure that the capacity within the community and academy exists to undertake community-based research? How do we continuously expose, question, and debate underlying values and assumptions? Community members might be resentful of us as academics because research is part of our job description. For community members, though, research participation is in addition to already heavy workloads and includes essentially volunteer work. How sustainable is community-based research when community members continuously engage in research as unpaid work?

Adding to the often complex and messy work in community-based research is the challenge of working with ethics review boards. While some ethics review boards have acknowledged the shifts necessary to support community-based research, other boards continue to operate within a bio-medical framework and focus on assessing risks to individual participants. When the focus is on individuals, the notion of community is lost, and risks to communities are neither acknowledged nor potentially assessed. Sarah Flicker and colleagues (2007) also point out that operating within a biomedical model continues "to perpetuate the notion that the domain of knowledge production is the sole right of academic researchers" (p. 478). The authors also argue that ethics review boards remain outsiders to communities and question the grounds on which ethics review boards assess risk and acceptability of the research. Can risk to a community or individual be assessed without knowing the community?

There is a danger that ethics review boards can silence communities, perpetuate social exclusion, and minimize the democratization of knowledge. "In some cases, ethical guidelines imposed by academic institutions morph into barriers to research; at other times, they overlap or stand in opposition to existing formal policies and informal practices in community agencies" (Ibáñez-Carrasco & Riano-Alcala, 2009, p. 85). While ethics review boards are important, it is critical to remember that community-based research is also about self-determination of communities, an important principle that researchers and communities must help ethics review boards understand. Involvement of community members at all stages of the research process is important, yet ethics review boards may see this as a threat to confidentiality and researcher control, which at times leads to abridged or superficial versions of community-based research (Stanton, 2014).

Contemplating Notions of Praxis

For us, one of the vital elements of community-based research is that we are part of the communities that participate in our research, but in ways that go beyond a *traditional* researcher role. In addition to our work as academics, both of us intentionally choose to be a part of communities. We have joined different agencies as volunteers, worked on boards of nonprofit agencies, become involved in community activities, and formed more longstanding friendships. Whereas research ethics boards ask researchers to adhere to a rigid understanding of personal and professional boundaries, we find ourselves in ongoing conversations about these boundaries with community members, students, and agencies. We often meet past and present collaborators and research participants at social functions, or past research participants contact us to continue conversations or see us as potentially helpful to their circumstances. For us, we never turn our backs to participants or community agencies in these encounters, but instead we engage in a process of renegotiating our relationships. This is important because we know that our paths will continue to cross as concerned citizens, friends, colleagues, or supervisors and mentors of students within and outside of the communities where we first met. Vera has been asked on several occasions to write letters of reference for community members or participants applying to universities or for jobs. As a result, we realize how important it is to see community-based research as relational engagement that must be continuously negotiated as well as a praxis.

For Patti Lather (1986), a commitment to praxis acknowledges "the critical and empowering roots of a research paradigm openly committed to critiquing the status quo and building a more just society" (p. 258). She argues that praxis-oriented research is about producing emancipatory knowledge while also empowering those who engage in research as participants. Like Lather, we do not see the commitment to praxis as a sign that we are turning away from empirical accountability. Instead, the involvement of the community in research must be balanced with agreed-upon methodologies and methods that make our empirical decisions transparent and accessible. In some of our projects we have come to know how significant it is to make our decisions visible, such as choosing particular methodologies or methods, setting inclusion and exclusion criteria for participants, and making transparent the multiple ways in which data are interpreted. For Mayan and Daum (2014), it is important that we critique the very same systems we have used.

As we think about praxis, we also are reminded how important it is to look at reward structures for all partners in community-based research, as well as strategies to sustain these partnerships. In our projects, we recognize that sustainability must be the focus of all team members and partners. To achieve sustainability, there must be a sense of a common goal and shared interest beyond individual research projects. The common goals may be achieved only in part through research. In our project on clinical mentorship in HIV care (Mill et al., 2014a), we worked closely with people living with HIV who provided mentorship to nurses inexperienced in HIV care. For them, the larger goal was to be recognized for their particular knowledge and for their ability to be involved in larger teaching initiatives. We were well aware that for many community members, teaching within the academy was seldom possible.

It is important to create spaces within universities where community members are welcomed. David Berg, whom we spoke about much earlier, was actively engaged in teaching undergraduate students in Vera's classrooms. Ray Chorney, with whom both Vera and Judy have worked closely in their research, and who sits on the board of directors for HIV Edmonton, worked with graduate students as they developed ideas for research. We also invite members from community agencies to be part of doctoral candidacy exams and final defense committees of graduate students. But we have faced many challenges because of our approach. For example, on one occasion we were questioned about the credentials of a staff member from a local AIDS service organization whom we wanted to be part of the supervisory committee for a doctoral student. Despite these challenges, we have seen the tremendous impact of community members on student learning and our ability to sustain and enrich partnerships with communities.

Another question that often troubles researchers is whether academic researchers should ensure that their research focus overlaps with their teaching and community service responsibilities. We say yes: academics have a responsibility to integrate their research, teaching, and community service. For example, Vera recently chaired the board of an inner-city agency that provides a range of services to many of the clients who participate in our research, while Judy was a member of the board of directors of HIV Edmonton for six years. In more recent times we have seen the spread of community service learning. This might be another way to not only create sustainability for long-term partnerships but also to ensure that community-based research is responsive to community needs. As Trussler and Marchand (2005) point out, community-based research "not only encourages critical reflectivity on the current state of things represented in data but also provides a structured format for organizational learning on the way to accomplishing humanly significant goals" (p. 46).

Criteria for Judging Quality

Though community-based research is not new, methodological issues regarding validity, reliability, and objectivity are still raised. Often these issues raise questions about the balance between scientific rigor and community acceptability (Horowitz et al., 2009). Ann Macaulay and colleagues (2011) also highlight several additional issues related to community-based research: difficulty assessing research quality, difficulty linking research quality to the quality of participatory elements, and difficulty attributing research outcomes to participation. We also notice these issues and realize that as researchers we have a responsibility to address these as we report on community-based research projects. Recently we have begun to write about research quality when doing community-based research. For example, following an international research program, Judy (Mill et al., 2014b) explored the challenges related to maintaining rigorous, high-quality research while building capacity. We also ask graduate students who engage in community-based research to develop methodological papers that address these issues as well as reflect the process of decision making and how these affect the findings, outcomes, and impacts of their studies. Perhaps we need to go beyond this, as others have pointed out that "[t]o the extent that [community-based participatory research] is seen as a process for enhancing community capacities, then it should be evaluated as a social intervention in itself" (Buchanan, Miller, & Wallerstein, 2007, p. 157).

Issues of rigor and validity need to be much more closely linked to relevance, whereby relevance is understood from multiple vantage points. In addition to standard forms of validity, such as face and construct validity, other ways to assess validity, such as social and cultural relevance, may need to be linked to community-based research to strengthen this approach. Patti Lather (1986) suggests catalytic validity as a way to represent "the degree to which the research process reorients, focuses, and energizes participants toward knowing reality in order to transform it, a process Freire (1973) terms conscientization" (p. 272).

Development of Jointly Agreed-upon Research Principles

In chapter 5 we talk at length about the importance of developing agreements that reflect research principles for each team and project; we return to this here. We emphasize research agreements because we have experienced disagreements and conflicts as well as deep divisions within the community itself and between the community and researchers about issues and processes. The process of developing these agreements is most important; often the issues become apparent when discussing how teams should work together. Having worked on multiple projects, we recognize that while some principles can be transferred between projects, "[e]very community is unique and may require a different approach or form of relationship" (Edwards et al., 2008, p. 192). While the significance of partnership and partnership agreements must be emphasized (Ross et al., 2010), agreements must also be written in ways that create flexibility and "honor the intention of shared responsibilities" (Green, 2004, p. 2).

Partnership agreements also need to recognize "how entangled academic-community relationships are . . . and embrac[e] the contradictions to confront power hierarchies of who tells the story or who creates knowledge" (Muhammad et al., 2014, p. 5). Muhammad and colleagues draw on social psychologist Michelle Fine's (1994) work to think about these entangled relationships, which Fine describes as "working the hyphen."

> By *working the hyphen*, I mean to suggest that researchers probe how we are in relation with the contexts we study and with our informants, understanding that we are all multiple in those relations. I mean to invite researchers to see how their "relations between" get us "better" data, limit what we feel free to say, expand our minds and constrict our mouth, engage us in intimacy and seduce us into complicity, make us quick to interpret and hesitant to write. Working the hyphen means creating occasions for researchers and informants to discuss what is, and is not, "happening between", within the negotiated relations of whose story is being told, why, to whom, with what interpretation, and whose story is shadowed, why, for whom, and with what consequence. (1994, p. 72; italics in original)

Fine points to key relational issues that require ongoing care, attention, and negotiation.

Proving Success, Shifting Inequities

Communities have a vested interest in community-based research, which provides an alternative approach to traditional research. Many community members and organizations see that traditional research does not shift the inequities they experience and that many of the disparities are actually increasing. Community-based research allows communities to be involved in identifying their most pressing issues and finding ways to inquire into them and propose evidence-informed interventions. For Trussler and Marchand (2005), community-based research "has shown that professional research and community inquiry are both knowledge construction in their own right, and both are necessary especially in light of what all knowledge is ultimately for: improvement of the human condition" (p. 46).

While success ultimately is considered the improvement of the human condition, how success or improvement is defined must be determined by the people and communities involved or potentially affected. It is important to define what success means while still remaining open to surprise and unanticipated outcomes. Judy has long worked with nurses and communities to take up notions of stigma in relation to HIV and AIDS. And while each of the projects had unique outcomes and impacts, stigma still remains a central issue for people living with HIV globally. By engaging communities to explore the impact, understandings, and implementation of interventions to reduce stigma, several outcomes reflect success within community-based research. First, the issue of stigma and discrimination is now central to conversations about HIV prevention, care and practice; second, the treatment of HIV as an *exceptional* disease may itself increase stigma, which is recognized within communities; and, finally, stigma reduction through particular interventions is possible but can be achieved only through the ongoing involvement of people living with HIV.

Both of us have been part of ongoing efforts to build capacity within communities to initiate and engage in community-based research. In addition, we have worked to build capacity in funding organizations and ethics review boards to assess and respond to community-based research. We have seen that attentive and involved partnerships between researchers situated in the academy, community members, and organizations can be synergistic and rewarding. In several of our projects we have also seen that the capacity to combine commitment with skepticism and inquiry engages the democratic spirit and is essential to democracy (Bateson, 1995). Community-based research can encourage those involved to ask new questions, develop different ideas, and challenge long-held assumptions and values.

In ongoing community-based research projects, it is important to explore the impact of participation not only on the substantive outcomes of a project but also on what difference participation makes to the life of the community. We also need to better understand the success of projects in relation to civic engagement (Stokamer, 2013), or personal engagement and growth as a result of participating in community-based research (Jacquez et al., 2013). Although we have anecdotal evidence of these effects, they require a more systematic inquiry and ultimately must be linked to potential long-term impacts that address inequities. Hacker and colleagues find that in community-based research:

(1) the concepts of capacity and sustainability were considered interconnected; (2) partnership was perceived as both a facilitator and an outcome of [community-based participatory research]; (3) sustainability was linked to "transfer of knowledge" from one generation to another within a community; and (4) capacity and sustainability were enhanced when goals were shared and health outcomes were achieved. (2012, p. 349)

As we write the final paragraph of this book, we think about our own beginnings in relation to community-based research. We find it difficult to decipher a clear beginning place; what we do know is that our work before becoming academics was strongly grounded in our experiences as community health nurses. Community-based research has allowed us to build on these early experiences, and has enabled us in our lives as academics to form profound relationships with practitioners and community members; to live in ways that, for us, speak to social justice; and to honor the relationships we have formed. We want to underline that community-based research is only one approach to research, and while this approach has worked well for us, it may not work for others. Ongoing challenges remain as we and others undertake this work together with people and practitioners in communities, but these challenges are also opportunities to learn, to push the boundaries of what research is and can be, and to democratize knowledge. Community-based research takes time and commitment. Perhaps it is only fitting at the end of this book to ask ourselves once more the question our friend David posed to us so many times: What are you waiting for?

Appendix: Resources on Community-based Research

This list of resources is a starting place to access additional information. Organizations that provide resources are primarily located in North America; some focus on international work. Many of the websites listed also link to additional resources; keep in mind that a variety of terms are used, including community-based research, community-based participatory research, and community-based participatory action research.

- **Community-Based Research Canada** (CBRC; http://communityresearchcanada.ca/) has a wide membership of academics and community organizations. Though based in Canada, CBRC has a strong link to a global network. Their key focus is on leading and supporting research and policy papers stemming from or focusing on community-based research.
- The **Community-Campus Partnerships for Health** (http://ccph.memberclicks.net) focuses on partnerships between communities and academic institutions. It is located in the United States and has a strong focus on training.
- The **University of Washington** (https://depts.washington.edu/ccph/cbpr/index.php) offers access to a well-developed curriculum for community-based research developed by leading scholars in the field.
- In 1982 the **Centre for Community-Based Research** (www.communitybasedresearch.ca/) was established, focused on linking research and education. The Centre emphasizes the use of social research to create inclusive communities.
- The **Arctic Institute of Community-Based Research** (www.aicbr.ca) is located in the Yukon and is focused on issues important to circumpolar regions. Both national and international partners are part of the larger network.
- Some websites focus on particular illnesses, such as HIV. **The Learning Place for CBR Research in HIV** (http://tlp.ohtn.on.ca) provides access to interactive learning modules and a connecting place for both communities and researchers.

Notes

Preface

1. Here we use first names to reflect the close relationship we had with David Berg. David gave us permission to talk about our experiences with him. He was a community advisory member for some of our work, and was also a friend and long-term AIDS activist.

Chapter 2

1. For a further discussion of community-based participatory research as an approach, see Flicker, 2008; Flicker et al., 2008b, 2008c, 2008d; Israel et al., 2005; Israel et al., 2006; Jacquez et al., 2013; Minkler, 2004, 2005; Minkler & Wallerstein, 2008; Nyden, 2003; Shore et al., 2008; Stanton, 2014.

2. For additional discussion about the challenges faced by community organizations to participate in research and at the same time provide service, see Flicker, 2008; Israel et al., 1998; Martz & Bacsu, 2014; Minkler & Wallerstein, 2008; Wallerstein & Duran, 2006.

3. The terms "Indigenous" and "Aboriginal" used in this book reflect the First Peoples of the world and Canada specifically. We use the term "Indigenous" when referring to broad, shared knowledge, values, and a world view reflective of our shared experiences and personal exchanges with other Indigenous researchers. We use the term "Aboriginal" when discussing the context of work specifically in Canada. Aboriginal Peoples is an umbrella term inclusive of First Nations, Inuit, and Métis, descendants of the original peoples of the territory that is now called Canada. For examples and further discussion of research with Indigenous communities, see Burhansstipanov, Christopher, & Schumacher, 2005; Fletcher, 2003; Macaulay et al., 1999; Marshall et al., 2014; Stanton, 2014; Strickland, 2006.

4. The following authors address the use of community-based research with populations and communities living with inequities: Flicker, 2008; Israel et al., 2006, 2008; Maclean, Warr, & Pyett, 2009; Minkler, 2005; Minkler & Wallerstein, 2008; Wallerstein & Duran, 2006.

Chapter 3

1. North Slavey consists of three different dialects. *Sahtúgot'ıné*, or Bear Slavey, as it was previously called, is spoken in Délįnę.

NOTES

Chapter 5

1. For examples and discussion of the development of Principles for Research Collaboration in community-based research see Flicker et al., 2007; Macaulay et al., 1999; Martz & Bacsu, 2014; Minkler, 2004; Ross et al., 2010.
2. Judy Mill would like to acknowledge the contributions of the members of the Partnership Task Group of the research program "Strengthening Nurses' Capacity for HIV Policy Development in sub-Saharan Africa and the Caribbean" (Edwards et al., 2013). These members had the responsibility for drafting principles for research collaboration for this international research program. This group included Josephine Etowa, Eulalia Kahwa, Susan Roelofs, and June Webber. We would also like to thank Nancy Edwards and Lynn McLean for their input on a previous version of this chapter.
3. At the University of Alberta, MOUs are agreements developed at the university level between the University of Alberta and international partner universities.
4. Barbados' participation in the research program ended in 2008.
5. For a discussion of the use of MOUs for community-based research, see Flicker, 2008; Martz & Bacsu, 2014; Minkler, 2004; Plumb et al., 2004; Ross et al., 2010.

Chapter 6

1. Several authors (Martz & Bacsu, 2014; Mikesell et al., 2013; Shore et al., 2008; Wallerstein & Duran, 2006) have argued that research ethics boards must assess the benefits and risks of the research from both an individual and community perspective.

Chapter 7

1. The concept of cultural humility has been discussed and advocated by several authors (Chavez et al., 2008; Fisher-Borne, Montana Cain, & Martin, 2014; Hockett, Samek, & Headley, 2014; Rhodes, 2014; Ross, 2010).

Chapter 8

1. See note 3 in chapter 2.
2. See Flicker et al. (2015), who describe the importance of Indigenous elders in community-based research.
3. Given the global cultural and knowledge diversity of Indigenous peoples, we purposefully use plural here as it is widely held by Indigenous and allied scholars that these knowledges are multiple.
4. OCAP™ has been trademarked by the First Nations Information Governance Centre. For more information, see www.fnigc.ca.

References

Ansari, W., Phillips, C., & Zwi, A. (2002). Narrowing the gap between academic professional wisdom and community lay knowledge: Perceptions from partnerships. *Public Health, 116*, 151–159.

Aveling, N. (2013). "Don't talk about what you don't know": On (not) conducting research with/in Indigenous contexts. *Critical Studies in Education, 54*(2), 203–214.

Balazs, C. L., & Morello-Frosch, R. (2013). The three Rs: How community-based participatory research strengthens the rigor, relevance, and reach of science. *Environmental Justice, 6*(1), 9–16.

Baldwin, J., Johnson, J., & Benally, C. (2009). Building partnerships between Indigenous communities and universities: Lessons learned in HIV/AIDS and substance abuse prevention research. *American Journal of Public Health, 99*(Suppl. 1), S77–S82.

Ball, J., & Janyst, P. (2008). Enacting research ethics in partnerships with Indigenous communities in Canada: "Do it in a good way". *Journal of Empirical Research on Human Research Ethics, 3*(2), 33–51.

Banks, S., Armstrong, A., Carter, K., Graham, H., Hayward, P., Henry, A., . . . Strachan, A. (2013). Everyday ethics in community based participatory research. *Contemporary Social Science: Journal of the Academy of Social Sciences, 8*(3), 263–277.

Barnes, H. (2000). Collaboration in community-action: A successful partnership between Indigenous communities and researchers. *Health Promotion International, 15*(1), 17–25.

Bateson, M. C. (1995). *Peripheral vision: Learning along the way*. New York: Perennial.

Benatar, S. R., & Singer, P. A. (2010). Responsibilities in international research: A new look revisited. *Journal of Medical Ethics, 36*(4), 194–197.

Bergum, V., & Dossetor, J. (2005). *Relational ethics: The full meaning of respect*. Hagerstown, MD: University Publishing Group.

Biesta, G. (2011). *Learning democracy in school and society: Education, lifelong learning, and the politics of citizenship*. Rotterdam, Netherlands: Sense Publisher.

Blodgett, A., Schinke, R., Peltier, D., Fisher, L., Watson, J., & Wabano, M. (2011). May the circle be unbroken: The research recommendations of Aboriginal community members engaged in participatory action research with university academics. *Journal of Sport and Social Issues, 35*(3), 264–283.

REFERENCES

Blow, P. (1998). *Village of widows.* [52 min., video]. Toronto, ON, Canada: Lindum Films.

Boyer, K., Orpin, P., & Walker, J. (2010). Partner or perish: Experiences from the field about collaborations for reform. *Australian Journal of Primary Health, 16,* 104–107.

Brant Castellano, M. (2000). Updating Aboriginal traditions of knowledge. In G. Sefa Dei, B. Hall, & D. Goldin Rosenburg (Eds.), *Indigenous knowledges in global contexts: Multiple readings of our world* (pp. 21–36). Toronto, ON, Canada: University of Toronto Press.

Braun, K., Browne, C., Ka'opua, L., Kim, B., & Mokuau, N. (2013). Research on Indigenous elders: From positivistic to decolonizing methodologies. *The Gerontologist, 54*(1), 117–126.

Brennan, D., Jackson, R., Zoccole, A., Nobis, A., Brett, C., & Georgievski, G. (2015). The seven truths of resilience: Understanding wellness and longevity among long-term HIV-positive gay, bisexual and Two-spirit males. Paper presented at the SSWR 19th Annual Conference: The Social and Behavioral Importance of Increased Longevity, New Orleans, LA: Society for Social Work and Research, January 14–18.

Browne, A., Smye, V., & Varcoe, C. (2005). The relevance of postcolonial theoretical perspectives to research in Aboriginal health. *Canadian Journal of Nursing Research, 37*(4), 16–37.

Brugge, D., & Missaghian, M. (2006). Protecting the Navajo people through tribal regulation of research. *Science and Engineering Ethics, 12,* 491–507.

Buchanan, D. R., Miller, F. G., & Wallerstein, N. (2007). Ethical issues in community based participatory research: Balancing rigorous research with community participation in community intervention studies. *Progress in Community Health Partnerships, 1*(2), 153–160.

Burhansstipanov, L., Christopher, S., & Schumacher, S. A. (2005). Lessons learned from community based participatory research in Indian country. *Cancer Control, 12*(Suppl. 2), 70–76.

Burke, J. G., Hess, S., Hoffmann, K., Guizzetti, L., Loy, E., Gielen, A., & Yonas, M. (2013). Translating community based participatory research principles into practice. *Progress in Community Health Partnerships: Research, Education, and Action, 7*(2), 115–122.

Burman, K. D. (1982). "Hanging from the masthead": Reflections on authorship. *Annals of Internal Medicine, 97,* 602–605.

Burnette, C., Sanders, S., Butcher, H., & Salois, E. (2011). Illuminating the lived experiences of research with Indigenous communities. *Journal of Ethnic & Cultural Diversity in Social Work, 20,* 275–296.

Cacari-Stone, L., Wallerstein, N., Garcia, A. P., & Minkler, M. (2014). The promise of community based participatory research for health equity: A conceptual model for bridging evidence with policy. *American Journal of Public Health, 104*(9), 1615–1623.

REFERENCES

Caine, K. J., Davison, C. M., & Stewart, E. J. (2009). Preliminary field-work: Methodological reflections from northern Canadian research. *Qualitative Research, 9*(4), 489–513.

Canadian Aboriginal AIDS Network (CAAN). (2010). *Negotiating ethical agreements.* Retrieved from http://caan.ca/new/wp-content/uploads/2010/06/Ethical%20Agreements.pdf

Canadian Coalition for Nuclear Responsibility. (1998, March 25). *The Dene people of Great Bear Lake call for a federal response to uranium deaths in Délı̨nę.* Retrieved from www.ccnr.org/dene.html

Canada-Délı̨nę Uranium Table (CDUT). (2005, August). *Canada-Déline uranium table final report: Concerning health and environmental issues related to the Port Radium Mine.* Déline, NT, Canada: Author.

Canadian Institutes of Health Research, Natural Sciences and Engineering Research Council of Canada, & Social Sciences and Humanities Research Council of Canada. (2010). *Tri-council policy statement: Ethical conduct for research involving humans.* Retrieved from www.pre.ethics.gc.ca/pdf/eng/tcps2/TCPS_2_FINAL_Web.pdf

Cargo, M., & Mercer, S. L. (2008). The value and challenges of participatory research: Strengthening its practice. *Annual Review of Public Health, 29,* 325–350.

Chang, C., Salvatore, A. L., Tau Lee, P., San Liu, S., Tom, A. T., Morales, A., . . . Minkler, M. (2013). Adapting to context in community-based participatory research: "Participatory starting point" in a Chinese Immigrant worker community. *American Journal of Community Psychology, 51*(3–4), 480–491.

Chavez, V., Duran, B., Baker, Q. E., Avila, M. M., & Wallerstein, N. (2008). The dance of race and privilege in community based participatory research. In M. Minkler & N. Wallerstein (Eds.), *Community based participatory research for health: From process to outcomes* (2nd ed.) (pp. 91–106). San Francisco, CA: Jossey-Bass.

Chung, K., & Lounsbury, D. W. (2006). The role of power, process, and relationships in participatory research for statewide HIV/AIDS programming. *Social Science & Medicine, 63*(8), 2129–2140.

Christensen, J. (2012). Telling stories: Exploring research storytelling as a meaningful approach to knowledge mobilization with Indigenous research collaborators and diverse audiences in community-based participatory research. *The Canadian Geographer, 56*(2), 231–242.

Clandinin, D. J., & Connelly, F. M. (2000). *Narrative inquiry: Experience and story in qualitative research.* San Francisco, CA: Jossey-Bass.

Coates, J., & Gray, M. (2006). An "Ecospiritual" perspective: Finally, a place for Indigenous approaches. *British Journal of Social Work, 36,* 381–399.

Cochran, P., Marshall, C., Garcia-Downing, C., Kendall, E., Cook, D., McCubbin, L., & Mariah, R. (2008). Indigenous ways of knowing: Implications for participatory research and community. *American Journal of Public Health, 98*(1), 22–27.

REFERENCES

Cohen, J. (2000). Balancing the collaboration equation. *Science, 288*(5474), 2155-2159.

Communitas. (2001-2005). In Douglas Harper (Ed.), *Online etymology dictionary.* Retrieved from www.etymonline.com/

Couzos, S., Lea, T., Culbong, M., & Culbong, M. (2005). "We are not just participants— we are in charge": The NACCHO ear trial and the process for Aboriginal community-controlled health research. *Ethnicity and Health, 10*(2), 91-111.

Crofoot Graham, T. (2002). Using reasons for living to connect to American Indian healing traditions. *Journal of Sociology & Social Welfare, 29*(1), 55-75.

Délı̨nę First Nations. (2005a). *If only we had known: The history of Port Radium as told by the Sahtúot'ine.* Calgary, AB, Canada: Friesens Press.

Délı̨nę First Nations. (2005b, June). *Dene ways of respecting the land and animal.* Délı̨nę, NT, Canada: Author.

Denzin, N. K. (1999). Two-stepping in the '90s. *Qualitative Inquiry, 5*(4), 568-572.

Denzin, N. K., & Lincoln, Y. S. (2005). *The handbook of qualitative research* (3rd ed.). Thousand Oaks, CA: Sage Publications.

DeSantis, G. (2014). Community based research and advocacy for change. In B. Jeffrey, I. M. Findlay, D. Martz, & L. Clarke (Eds.), *Journey in community based research* (pp. 53-72). Regina, SK, Canada: University of Regina Press.

Dewey, J. (1916). *Democracy and education.* New York: MacMillan.

Drevdahl, D. J. (2002). Home and border: The contradictions of community. *Advances in Nursing Science, 24*(3), 8-20.

Du Bois, W. E. B. (1903). *The Souls of Black Folk.* Chicago, IL: A. C. McClurg.

Dunbar, T., & Scrimgeour, M. (2006). Ethics in Indigenous research: Connecting with community. *Bioethical Inquiry, 3*, 179-185.

Edwards, K., Lund, C., Mitchell, S., & Andersson, N. (2008). Trust the process: Community based researcher partnerships. *Pimatisiwin: A Journal of Aboriginal and Indigenous Community Health, 6*(2), 187-199.

Edwards, N., Kahwa, E., Kaseje, D., Mill, J., Webber, J., & Roelofs, S. (2007). Strengthening health care systems for HIV and AIDS in sub-Saharan Africa and the Caribbean: A programme of research. *The Caribbean Journal of Nursing & Midwifery, 2*, 29-36.

Etmanski, C., Hall, B. L., & Sawson, T. (Eds.). (2014). *Learning and teaching community-based research.* Toronto, ON, Canada: University of Toronto Press.

Etowa, J., Bernard, W. T., Oyinsan, B., & Clow, B. (2007). Participatory action research: An approach for improving Black women's health in rural and remote communities. *Journal of Transcultural Nursing, 18*(4), 349-357.

Evans, M., Hole, R., Berg, L., Hutchinson, P., & Sookraj, D. (2009). Common insights, differing methodologies: Toward a fusion of indigenous methodologies, participatory action research, and White studies in an urban Aboriginal research agenda. *Qualitative Inquiry, 15*(5), 893-910.

Fals-Borda, O., & Rahman, M. A. (1991). *Action and knowledge: Breaking the monopoly with participatory action research.* New York: APEX Press.

REFERENCES

Fawcett, S. B., Francisco, V. T., Paine-Andrews, A., & Schultz, J. A. (2000). A model memorandum of collaboration: A proposal. *Public Health Reports, 115,* 174–179.

Fine, M. (1994). Working the hyphens: Reinventing self and other in qualitative research. In N. K. Denzin & Y. S. Lincoln (Eds.), *Handbook of qualitative research* (pp. 70–82). Thousand Oaks, CA: Sage Publications.

Fisher-Borne, M., Montana Cain, J., & Martin, S. L. (2015). From mastery to accountability: Cultural humility as an alternative to cultural competence. *Social Work Education: The International Journal, 34*(2), 165–181.

Fletcher, C. (2003). Community based participatory research relationships with aboriginal communities in Canada: An overview of context and process. *Pimatisiwin: A Journal of Aboriginal & Indigenous Community Health, 1*(1), 27–61.

Flicker, S. (2008). Who benefits from community based participatory research? A case study of a positive youth project. *Health Education & Behaviour, 35*(1), 70–86.

Flicker, S., Larkin, J., Smilie-Adjarkwa, C., Restoule, J., Barlow, K., Dagnino, M., . . . Mitchell, C. (2008c). "It's hard to change something when you don't know where to start": Unpacking HIV vulnerability with Aboriginal youth in Canada. *Pimatisiwin: A Journal of Aboriginal and Indigenous Community Health, 5*(2), 175–200.

Flicker, S., & Nixon, S. (2014). The DEPICT model for participatory qualitative health promotion research analysis piloted in Canada, Zambia and South Africa. *Health Promotion International,* Prepublished online January 14 (most recently published August 2015). Retrieved from http://heapro.oxfordjournals.org/content/early/2014/01/12/heapro.dat093.full

Flicker, S., O'Campo, P., Monchalin, R., Thistle, J., Worthington, C., Masching, R., . . . Thomas, C. (2015). Research done in "A good way": The importance of indigenous elder involvement in HIV community-based research. *American Journal of Public Health, 105*(6), 1149–1154.

Flicker, S., Savan, B., Kolenda, B., & Mildenberger, M. (2008b). A snapshot of community based research in Canada: Who? What? Why? How?. *Health Education Research, 23*(1), 106–114.

Flicker, S., Savan, B., McGrath, M., Kolenda, B., & Mildenberger, M. (2008a). "If you could change one thing . . .": What community based researchers wish they could have done differently. *Community Development Journal, 43*(2), 239–253.

Flicker, S., Travers, R., Guta, A., McDonald, S., & Meagher, A. (2007). Ethical dilemmas in community based participatory research: Recommendations for institutional review boards. *Journal of Urban Health, 84*(4), 478–493.

Freire, P. (1973). *Education for critical consciousness.* New York: Continuum.

Freire, P. (1989/1968). *Pedagogy of the oppressed.* (Trans. M. B. Ramos). New York: The Continuum Publishing Company.

Freudenberg, N., & Tsui, E. (2014). Evidence, power, and policy change in community based participatory research. *American Journal of Public Health, 104*(1), 11–14.

REFERENCES

Gamble, V. N., & Stone, D. (2006). U. S. policy on health inequities: The interplay of politics and research. *Journal of Health Politics, Policy and Law, 31*(1), 93–126.

Garcia, A. P., Minkler, M., Cardenas, Z., Grills, C., & Porter, C. (2014). Engaging homeless youth in community based participatory research: A case study from skid row, Los Angeles. *Health Promotion Practice, 15*(1), 18–27.

George, C., Adam, B. A., Stanley, S. E., Husbands, W. C., Remis, R. S., Makoroka, L., & Rourke, S. B. (2012). The MaBwana men's study: Community and belonging in the lives of African, Caribbean and other black gay men in Toronto. *Culture, Health & Sexuality, 24*(5), 549–562.

Getty, G. (2010). The journey between western and Indigenous research paradigms. *Journal of Transcultural Nursing, 21*(1), 5–14.

Giroux, H. (2003). Democracy, patriotism and schooling after September 11: Critical citizens or unthinking patriots. In H. Giroux (Ed.), *The abandoned generation: Democracy beyond the culture of fear* (pp. 16–45). New York: Palgrave MacMillan.

Green, L., Daniel, M., & Novick, L. (2001). Partnership and coalitions for community-based research. *Public Health Report, 116*(Suppl. 1), 20–31.

Green, L. W. (2004). Ethics and community based participatory research: Commentary on Minkler. *Health Education & Behavior, 31*(6), 1–4.

Greene, M. (1995). *Releasing the imagination: Essays on education, the arts, and social change.* San Francisco, CA: Jossey-Bass.

Grieger, M. C. A. (2005). Authorship: An ethical dilemma of science. *Sao Paulo Medical Journal, 123*(5), 242–246.

Guta, A., Flicker, S., & Roche, B. (2013a). Governing through community allegiance: A qualitative examination of peer research in community-based participatory research. *Critical Public Health, 23*(4), 432–452.

Guta, A., Nixon, S., & Wilson, M. G. (2013b). Resisting the seduction of "ethics creep": Using Foucault to surface complexity and contradiction in research ethics review. *Social Science & Medicine, 98*, 301–310.

Hacker, K., Tendulkar, S. A., Rideout, C., Bhuiya, N., Trinh-Shevrin, C., Savage, C. P., . . . DiGirolamo, A. M. (2012). Community capacity building and sustainability: Outcomes of community-based participatory research. *Progress in Community Health Partnerships: Research, Education, and Action, 6*(3), 349–360.

Hall, B. (1981). Participatory research, popular knowledge, and power: A personal reflection. *Convergence, 14*(3), 6–17.

Hall, B. (1988). The democratization of the production of knowledge. Paper presented at the University of Leeds, England.

Hall, B. (1993). Introduction. In P. Park, M. Brydon-Miller, B. Hall, & T. Jackson (Eds.), *Voices of change: Participatory research in the United States and Canada* (pp. xiii–xxii). Toronto, ON, Canada: OISE Press.

Harrowing, J., Mill, J., Spiers, J., Kulig, J., & Kipp, W. (2010). Culture, context, and community: Ethical considerations for global nursing research. *International Nursing Review, 57*, 70–77.

REFERENCES

Hart, M. (2010). Indigenous worldviews, knowledge, and research: The development of an Indigenous research paradigm. *Journal of Indigenous Voices in Social Work, 1*(1), 1–16.

Hatcher, A., & Bartlett, C. (2010, May). Two-eyed seeing: Building cultural bridges for Aboriginal students. *Canadian Teacher Magazine, 6*(5), 14–17.

Heffner, G. G., Zandee, G. L., & Schwander, L. (2003). Listening to community voices: Community based research, a first step in partnership and outreach. *Journal of Higher Education Outreach and Engagement, 8*(1), 127–139.

Hockett, E., Samek, L., & Headley, S. (2014). Cultural humility: A framework for local and global engagement. *George Fox University faculty publications—School of Education* paper 13. Retrieved from http://digitalcommons.georgefox.edu/soe_faculty/13

Horowitz, C. R., Robinson, M., & Seifer, S. (2009). Community based participatory research from the margin to the mainstream: Are researchers prepared? *Circulation, 119*(19), 2633–2642.

Hunter, R., Liese, H., Burns, K., & Mai, T. (2011). Art and social justice: An interdisciplinary framework for community based teaching and research. *The International Journal of Higher Education and Democracy, 2*, 48–62.

Huth, E. J. (1986). Guidelines on authorship of medical papers. *Annals of Internal Medicine, 104*, 269–274.

Ibáñez-Carrasco, F. (2004). Desire and betrayal in community-based research. In F. Ibáñez-Carrasco & E. R. Meiners (Eds.), *Public acts: Disruptive readings on making curriculum public* (pp. 35–56). New York: Routledge Falmer.

Ibáñez-Carrasco, F., & Riano-Alcala, P. (2009). Organizing community-based research knowledge between universities and communities: Lessons learned. *Community Development Journal, 46*(1), 72–88.

International Committee of Medical Journal Editors (ICMJE). (1985). Guidelines on Authorship. *British Medical Journal, 291*, 722.

International Committee of Medical Journal Editors (ICMJE). (1993). Uniform requirements for manuscripts submitted to biomedical journals. *Journal of the American Medical Association, 269*(17), 2282–2286.

International Committee of Medical Journal Editors (ICMJE). (2009). *Uniform requirements for manuscripts submitted to biomedical journals.* Retrieved from www.icmje.org/ethical_1author.html

Israel, B., Coombe, C., Cheezum, R., Schulz, A., McGranaghan, R., Lichtenstein, R., . . . Burris, A. (2010). Community-based participatory research: a capacity building approach for policy advocacy aimed at eliminating health disparities. *American Journal of Public Health, 100*, 2094–2102.

Israel, B., Eng, E., Schulz, A., & Parker, E. (2005). *Methods in community based participatory research for health.* San Francisco, CA: John Wiley & Sons.

Israel, B. A., Krieger, J., Vlahov, D., Ciske, S., Foley, M., Fortin, P., . . . Tang, G. (2006). Challenges and facilitating factors in sustaining community based participatory research partnerships: Lessons learned from the Detroit, New York

REFERENCES

City and Seattle urban research centers. *Journal of Urban Health, 83*(6), 1022–1040.

Israel, B. A., Schulz, A. J., Parker, E. A., & Becker, A. B. (1998). Review of community based research: Assessing partnership approaches to improve public health. *Annual Review of Public Health, 19*, 173–202.

Israel, B. A., Schulz, A. J., Parker, E. A., Becker, A. B., Allen, A. J., & Guzman, R. (2008). Critical issues in developing and following CBPR principles. In M. Minkler & N. Wallerstein (Eds.), *Community based participatory research for health: From process to outcomes* (2nd ed.) (pp. 47–66). San Francisco, CA: Jossey-Bass.

Iwama, M., Marshall, M., Marshall, A., & Bartlett, C. (2009). Two-eyed seeing and the language of healing in community-based research. *Canadian Journal of Native Education, 32*(2), 3–23.

Jacklin, K., & Kinoshameg, P. (2008). Developing a participatory Aboriginal health research project: "Only if it's going to mean something." *Journal of Empirical Research of Human Research Ethics, 3*(2), 53–68.

Jackson, R., Debassige, C., Masching, R., & Whitebird, W. (2014). Towards an Indigenous narrative inquiry: The importance of composite, artful representations. In C. Sinding & H. Barnes (Eds.), *Social work artfully: Beyond borders and boundaries* (pp. 135–158). Waterloo, ON, Canada: Wilfrid Laurier Press.

Jackson, R., Dixon, L., Thomas, K., & Zoccole, A. (2003, April). One example of negotiating a research partnership. Paper presented at the Canadian Association for AIDS Research Conference, Halifax, NS, Canada, April 10–13.

Jackson, S. (2008). A participatory group process to analyze qualitative data. *Progress in Community Health Partnerships: Research, Education and Action, 2*(2), 161–170.

Jacquez, F., Vaughn, L. M., & Wagner, E. (2013). Youth as partners, participants or passive recipients: A review of children and adolescents in community-based participatory research (CBPR). *American Journal of Community Psychology, 51*, 176–189.

Jagosh, J., Macaulay, A. C., Pluye, P., Salsberg, J., Bush, P. L., Henderson, J., . . . & Greenhalgh, T. (2012). Uncovering the benefits of participatory research: Implications of a realist review for health research and practice. *Milbank Quarterly, 90*(2), 311–346.

Joint United Nations Programme on HIV/AIDS (UNAIDS). (1999). *From principle to practice: Greater involvement of people living with or affected by HIV/AIDS (GIPA)*. Geneva, Switzerland: Van Roey, J.

Jolivette, A. (2015). *Research justice: Methodologies for social change*. Chicago, IL: University of Chicago Press.

Jones, A., & Jenkins, K. (2008). Rethinking collaboration: Working the indigene-colonizer hyphen. In N. Denzin, Y. Lincoln, & L. Smith (Eds.), *Handbook of critical and Indigenous methodologies* (pp. 471–486). Thousand Oaks, California: Sage Publications.

REFERENCES

Jones, L., & Wells, K. (2007). Strategies for academic and clinician engagement in community-participatory partnered research. *Journal of the American Medical Association, 297*(4), 407–410.

Kaplan-Myrth, N., & Smylie, J. (2006). *Sharing what we know about living a good life: Indigenous knowledge translation summit.* Regina, SK, Canada: First Nations University of Canada.

Katz, J. S., & Martin, B. R. (1997). What is research collaboration? *Research Policy, 26,* 1–18.

Kaufert, J., Commanda, L., Elias, B., Grey, R., Masuzumi, B., & Young, K. (2001). Community participation in health research ethics. In J. Oakes, R. Riewe, M. Bennett, & B. Chisholm (Eds.), *Pushing the margins: Narrative and northern studies* (pp. 50–61). Winnipeg, MB, Canada: Native Studies Press.

Kellogg Foundation. (2015). *Community track training sites.* Retrieved from www.kellogghealthscholars.org/sites/community.php

Kendall, E., Sunderland, N., Barnett, L., Nalder, G., & Matthews, C. (2011). Beyond the rhetoric of participatory research in Indigenous communities: Advances in Australia over the last decade. *Qualitative Health Research, 21*(12), 1719–1728.

Kincheloe, J., & Steinberg, S. (2008). Indigenous knowledges in education: Complexities, dangers, and profound benefits. In N. Denzin, Y. Lincoln, & L. Smith (Eds.), *Handbook of critical and Indigenous methodologies* (pp. 135–156). Thousand Oaks, California: Sage Publications.

Kingsley, B. C., & Chapman, S. A. (2013). Questioning the meaningfulness of rigour in community-based research: Navigating a dilemma. *International Journal of Qualitative Methods, 12,* 551–569.

Kirkness, V. J., & Barnhard, R. (2001). First Nations and higher education: The four R's—espect, relevance, reciprocity, responsibility. In R. Hayoe & J. Pam (Eds.), *Knowledge across cultures: A contribution to dialogue among civilizations* (pp. 75–91). Hong Kong: Comparative Education Research Centre, University of Hong Kong.

Koster, R., Baccar, K., & Lemelin, H. (2012). Moving from research ON, to research WITH and FOR Indigenous communities: A critical reflection on community-based participatory research. *The Canadian Geographer, 56*(2), 195–210.

Lasker, R. D., & Weiss, E. S. (2003). Creating partnership synergy: The critical role of community stakeholders. *Journal of Health and Human Service Administration, 26*(1), 119–139.

Lasker, R. D., Weiss, E. S., & Miller, R. (2001). Partnership synergy: A practical framework for studying and strengthening the collaborative advantage. *The Millbank Quarterly, 79*(2), 179–205.

Lather, P. (1986). Research as praxis. *Harvard Educational Review, 56*(3), 257–277.

Lather, P. (2013). Methodology-21: What do we do in the afterward? *International Journal of Qualitative Studies in Education, 26*(6), 634–645.

REFERENCES

Leash, E. (2010). Is it time for a new approach to authorship? *Council of Science Editors*. Retrieved from www.councilscienceeditors.org/i4a/pages/index.dfm? pageid=3408

Lewin, K. (1946). Action research and minority problems. *Journal of Social Issues, 2*, 34–46.

Lincoln, Y., & Denzin, N. (2008). Epilogue: The lion speaks. In N. Denzin, Y. Lincoln, & L. Smith (Eds.), *Handbook of critical and Indigenous methodologies* (pp. 563–571). Thousand Oaks, CA: Sage Publications.

Loewenson, R., Laurell, A. C., Hogstedt, C., D'Ambruoso, L., & Shroff, Z. (2014). *Participatory action research in health systems: A methods reader.* Harare, Zimbabwe: TARSC, AHPSR, WHO, IDRC Canada, EQUINET.

London, J. K. (2007). Power and pitfalls of youth participation in community based action research. *Children, Youth and Environments, 17*(2), 406–432.

Macaulay, A. C., Commanda, L. E., Freeman, W. L., Gibson, N., McCabe, M. L., Robbins, C. M., & Twohig, P. L. (1999). Participatory research maximises community and lay involvement. *British Medical Journal, 319*(7212), 774–778.

Macaulay, A. C., Jagosh, J., Seller, R., Henderson, J., Cargo, M., Greenhalgh, T., . . . Pluye, P. (2011). Assessing the benefits of participatory research: A rationale for a realist review. *Global Health Promotion, 18*(2), 45–48.

Macaulay, A. C., & Nutting, P. A. (2006). Moving the frontiers forward: Incorporating community based participatory research into practice-based research networks. *Annals of Family Medicine, 4*(1), 4–7.

MacLean, S., Warr, D., & Pyett, P. (2009). Was it good for you too? Impediments to conducting university-based collaborative research with communities experiencing disadvantage. *Australian and New Zealand Journal of Public Health, 33*(5), 407–412.

Maiter, S., Simich, L., Jacobson, N., & Wise, J. (2008). Reciprocity: An ethic for participatory action research with culturally diverse communities. *Action Research, 6*(3), 305–325.

Manson, S., Garroutte, E., Goins, R., & Henderson, P. (2004). Access, relevance, and control in the research process: Lessions from Indian country. *Journal of Aging and Health, 16*(5), 58S–77S.

Markey, A. (2005, September 12). Délįnę uranium report released. *Northern News Services*. Retrieved from www.nnsl.com/frames/newspapers/2005-09/sep12_05rad.html

Marshall, E. A., Peterson, R., Coverdale, J., Etzel, S., & McFarland, N. (2014). Learning and living community based research: Graduate student collaborations in Aboriginal communities. In B. Hall, C. Etmanski, & T. Dawson (Eds.), *Learning and teaching community based research: Linking pedagogy to practice.* (pp. 206–229). Toronto, ON, Canada: University of Toronto Press.

Martz, D., & Bacsu, J. (2014). Working together: Ethical practice in community-engaged research. In B. Jeffrey, I. M. Findlay, D. Martz, & L. Clarke (Eds.),

Journey in community based research (pp. 3–14). Regina, SK, Canada: University of Regina Press.

Marullo, S. Cooke, D., Willis, J., Rollins, A., Burke, J., Bonilla, P., & Waldref, V. (2003). Community-based research assessments: Some principles and practices. *Michigan Journal of Community Service Learning, 9*(3), np.

Masching, R. (2006). *Researching ourselves to life: Strategic research priorities, the CBR process & knowledge translation* [internal document]. Ottawa, ON, Canada: CAAN.

Masching, R., Allard, Y., & Prentice, T. (2006). Knowledge translation and Aboriginal HIV/AIDS research: Methods at the margins. *Canadian Journal of Aboriginal Community-based HIV/AIDS Research, 1*, 31–44.

Mayan, M., & Daum, C. (2014). Politics and public policy, social justice, and qualitative research. In N. K. Norman & M. D. Giardina (Eds.), *Qualitative inquiry outside the academy* (pp. 73–91). Walnut Creek, CA: Left Coast Press, Inc.

McLaren, P. (1989). *Life in schools: An introduction to critical pedagogy in the foundations of education.* New York: Longman.

McLeod, N. (2007). *Cree narrative memory: From treaties to contemporary rime.* Saskatoon, SK, Canada: Purich Publishing Ltd.

Meiners, E. R. (2004). Working between university and community: Shifting the focus, shifting the practice. In F. Ibáñez-Carrasco & E. R. Meiners (Eds.), *Public acts: Disruptive readings on making curriculum public* (pp. 161–180). New York: Routledge Falmer.

Mikesell, L., Bromley, E., & Khodyakov, D. (2013). Ethical community-engaged research: A literature review. *American Journal of Public Health, 103*(12), e7–e14.

Mill, J. E. (2003). Shrouded in secrecy: Breaking the news of HIV infection to Ghanaian women. *Journal of Transcultural Nursing, 14*(1), 6–16.

Mill, J. E., & Anarfi, J. K. (2002). HIV risk environment for Ghanaian women: Challenges to prevention. *Social Science and Medicine, 54*, 325–337.

Mill, J., Caine, V., Arneson, C., Maina, G., dePadua, T., & Dykeman, M. (2014a). Past experiences, current realities and future possibilities for HIV nursing education and care in Canada. *Journal of Nursing Education and Practice, 4*(5), 183–198.

Mill, J., Davison, C., Richter, S., Etowa, J., Edwards, N., Kahwa, E., . . . Harrowing, J. (2014b). Qualitative research in an international research program: Maintaining momentum while building capacity in nurses. *International Journal of Qualitative Methods, 13*, 151–169.

Mill, J., Edwards, N., Jackson, R., Austin, W., Maclean, L., & Reintjes, F. (2009). Accessing health services while living with HIV: Intersections of stigma. *Canadian Journal of Nursing Research, 41*(3), 168–185.

Mill, J., Jackson, R., Worthington, C. A., Archibald, C., Wong, T., Myers, T., . . . Sommerfeldt, S. (2008). HIV testing and care in Canadian Aboriginal youth: A community based mixed methods study. *BMC Infectious Diseases, 8*, 132–145.

REFERENCES

Mill, J., Lambert, D., Larkin, K., Ward, K., & Harrowing, J. (2007). Challenging lifestyles: Aboriginal men and women living with HIV. *Pimatisiwin: A Journal of Indigenous and Aboriginal Community Health, 5*(2), 151–173.

Mill, J., Singh, A., & Taylor, M. (2012). Women in the shadows: Prenatal care for street-involved women. *Canadian Journal of Urban Research, 21*(2), 68–89.

Mill, J. E., & Ogilvie, L. D. (2002). Ethical decision-making in international nursing research. *Qualitative Health Research, 12*(6), 807–815.

Minkler, M. (2004). Ethical challenges for the "outside" researcher in community based participatory research. *Health Education and Behaviour, 31*(6), 684–697.

Minkler, M. (2005). Community based research partnerships: Challenges and opportunities. *Journal of Urban Health, 82*(Suppl. 2), ii3–ii12.

Minkler, M. (2010). Linking science and policy through community based participatory research to study and address health disparities. *American Journal of Public Health, 100*(Suppl. 1), S81–S87.

Minkler, M., Blackwell, A. G., Thompson, M., & Tamir, H. (2003). Community based participatory research: Implications for public health funding. *American Journal of Public Health, 93*(8), 1210–1213.

Minkler, M., & Wallerstein, N. (Eds.). (2008). *Community-based participatory research for health: From process to outcomes.* San Francisco, CA: John Wiley & Sons.

Muhammad, M., Wallerstein, N., Sussman, A. L., Avila, M., Belone, L., & Duran, B. (2014). Reflections on research identity and power: The impact of positionality on community based participatory research (CBPR) processes and outcomes. *Critical Sociology,* Prepublished online May 30. Retrieved from http://crs.sagepub.com/content/early/2014/06/11/0896920513516025.abstract

Nyden, P. (2003). Academic incentives for faculty participation in community based participatory research. *Journal of General Internal Medicine, 18*(7), 576–585.

Oakley, A. (1981). Interviewing women: A contradiction in terms. In H. Roberts (Ed.), *Doing feminist research* (pp. 30–61). Boston, MA: Routledge & Kegan Paul.

O'Brien, M. J., & Whitaker, R. C. (2011). The role of community based participatory research to inform local health policy: A case study. *Journal of General Internal Medicine, 26*(12), 1498–1501.

Onyancha, O. B., & Ocholla, D. N. (2007). Country-wide collaborations in HIV/ AIDS research in Kenya and South Africa, 1980–2005. *Libri, 57,* 239–254.

Ordonez-Matamoros, H. G., Cozzens, S. E., & Garcia, M. (2009). International co-authorship and research team performance in Columbia. *Review of Policy Research, 27*(4), 415–431.

Paszek, T. (2012). *Educating for democratic citizenship: A narrative inquiry into teacher experiences* (Doctoral dissertation). Retrieved from University of Alberta Library institutional repository (uac.50814c9d.44a8.406b.a1c4.4e75ad67d3ea)

Patterson, M., Jackson, R., & Edwards, N. (2006). Ethics in Aboriginal research: Comments on paradigms, process and two worlds. *Canadian Journal of Aboriginal Community based HIV/AIDS Research, 1*(Summer), 47–61.

REFERENCES

Peltier, D., Jackson, R., Prentice, T., Masching, R., Fong, M., & Shore, K. (2011). *Supporting Aboriginal women involvement: An example of writing using community-based research principles.* Toronto, ON, Canada: Canadian Association of HIV Research.

Plumb, M., Price, W., & Kavanaugh-Lynch, M. H. (2004). Funding community based participatory research: Lessons learned. *Journal of Interprofessional Care, 18*(4), 428–439.

Respect. (2001–2005). In Douglas Harper (Ed.), *Online etymology dictionary.* Retrieved from www.etymonline.com/

Rhodes, S. (2014). Authentic community engagement and community-based participatory research for public health and medicine. In S. D. Rhodes (Ed.), *Innovations in HIV prevention research and practice through community engagement* (pp. 1–10). New York: Springer.

Richter, S., Mill, J., Muller, C. E., Kahwa, E., Etowa, J., Dawkins, P., & Hepburn, C. (2013). Nurses' engagement in AIDS policy development. *International Nursing Review, 60*(1), 52–58.

Ritchie, S. D., Jo Wabano, M., Beardy, J., Curran, J., Orkin, A., VandeBurgh, D., & Young, N. L. (2013). Community-based participatory research with indigenous communities: The proximity paradox. *Health Place, 24*, 183–189.

Ross, L. (2010). Notes from the field: Learning cultural humility through critical incidents and central challenges in community-based participatory research. *Journal of Community Practice, 18*(2–3), 315–335.

Ross, L. F., Loup, A., Nelson, R. M., Botkin, J. R., Kost, R., Smith, G. R., & Gehlert, S. (2010). The challenges of collaboration for academic and community partners in a research partnership: Points to consider. *Journal of Empirical Research on Human Research Ethics: An international Journal, 5*(1), 19–31.

Savan, B., Flicker, S., Kolenda, B., & Mildenberger, M. (2009). How to facilitate (or discourage) community-based research: Recommendations based on a Canadian survey. *Local Environment, 14*(8), 783–796.

Scarinci, I. C., Johnson, R. E., Hardy, C., Marron, J., & Partridge, E. E. (2009). Planning and implementation of a participatory evaluation strategy: A viable approach in the evaluation of community-based participatory programs addressing cancer disparities. *Evaluation of Program Panning, 32*(2), 221–228.

Schiltz, A., & Sandfort, G. (2000). HIV-positive people, risk, and sexual behavior. *Social Science and Medicine, 50*, 1571–1588.

Schnarch, B. (2004). Ownership, control, access, and possession (OCAP) or self-determination applied to research. *Journal of Aboriginal Health, 1*(1), 80–95.

Seifer, S. D. (2008). Making the best case for community-engaged scholarship in promotion and tenure review. In M. Minkler & N. Wallerstein (Eds.), *Community based participatory research for health* (pp. 425–430). San Francisco, CA: John Wiley & Sons.

Sernak, K. (2009). Dewey, democratic leadership, and art. In P. Jenlink (Ed.), *Dewey's democracy and education revisited: Contemporary discourses for democratic education and leadership* (pp. 163–186). Lanham, MD: Rowman & Littlefield Education.

Sherwood, J., & Edwards, T. (2006). Decolonisation: A critical step for improving Aboriginal health. *Contemporary Nurse, 22,* 178–190.

Shore, N., Wong, K. A., Seifer, S. D., Grignon, J., & Gamble, V. N. (2008). Introduction to special issue: Advancing the ethics of community based participatory research. *Journal of Empirical Research on Human Research Ethics, 3*(2), 1–4.

Simon, R. (2001). Now's the time. In J. Portelli & R. P. Solomon (Eds.), *The erosion of democracy in education* (pp. 11–13). Calgary, AB, Canada: Detselig Enterprises Ltd.

Smith, A., Christopher, S., & McCormick, A. (2004). Development and implementation of a cultural sensitive cervical health survey: A community-based participatory approach. *Women & Health, 40*(2), 67–86.

Smith, L. (1999). *Decolonizing methodologies: Research and Indigenous peoples.* New York: Zed Books Ltd.

Springett, J., Wright, M. T., & Roche, B. (2011). *Developing quality criteria for participatory health research: An agenda for action* (Discussion paper SP I 2011-302). Berlin, Germany: Social Science Center Berlin (WZB). Retrieved from http://bibliothek.wzb.eu/pdf/2011/i11-302.pdf

Stanton, C. R. (2014). Crossing methodological borders: Decolonizing community based participatory research. *Qualitative Inquiry, 20*(5), 573–583.

Stoecker, R. (2008). Are academics irrelevant? Approaches and roles for scholars in community-based research. In M. Minkler & N. Wallerstein (Eds.), *Community based participatory research for health: From process to outcomes* (2nd ed.) (pp. 107–120). San Francisco, CA: Jossey-Bass.

Stokamer, S. (2013). Pedagogical catalysts of civic competence: The development of a critical epistemological model for community-based learning. *Journal of Higher Education Outreach and Engagement, 17*(1), 113–121.

Strand, K., Marullo, S., Cutforth, N., Stoecker, R., & Donohue, P. (2003). Principles of best practice for community based research. *Michigan Journal of Community Service Learning, 9*(3), 5–15.

Strickland, C. J. (2006). Challenges in community based participatory research implementation: Experiences in cancer prevention in Pacific Northwest American tribes. *Cancer Control, 13*(3), 230–236.

Tedlock, B. (2011). Braiding narrative enthnography with memoir and creative nonfiction. In N. Denzin & Y. Lincoln (Eds.), *Handbook of qualitative research* (4th ed.) (pp. 331–339). Thousand Oaks, CA: Sage Publications.

Tervalon, M., & Murray-Garcia, J. (1998). Cultural humility versus cultural competence: A critical distinction in defining physician training outcomes in multicultural education. *Journal of Health Care for the Poor and Underserved, 9*(2), 117–125.

Themba-Nixon, M., Minkler, M., & Freudenberg, N. (2008). The role of community-based research in policy advocacy. In M. Minkler & N. Wallerstein

REFERENCES

(Eds.), *Community based participatory research for health: From process to outcomes* (2nd ed.) (pp. 307–322). San Francisco, CA: John Wiley & Sons.

Trussler, T., & Marchand, R. (2005). HIV/AIDS community based research. *New Directions for Adult and Continuing Education, 105*(Spring), 43–54.

van de Sande, A., & Schwartz, K. (2011). *Research for social justice: A community based approach.* Black Point, NS, Canada: Fernwood Publishing.

van Wyck, P. (2010). *The highway of the atom.* Montreal, QC, Canada: McGill-Queen's University Press.

Viswanathan, M., Ammerman, A., Eng, E., Gartlehner, G., Lohr, K. N., Griffith, D., . . . Whitener, L. (2004). *Community-based participatory research: Assessing the evidence.* Evidence Report/Technology Assessment No. 99 (Prepared by RTI–University of North Carolina Evidence-based Practice Center under Contract No. 290-02-0016). AHRQ Publication 04-E022-2. Rockville, MD: Agency for Healthcare Research and Quality.

Vogel, I. (2011). *Research capacity strengthening: Learning from experience.* Report from the UK Collaborative on Development Series. Retrieved from www.ukcds.org.uk/sites/default/files/content/resources/UKCDS_Capacity_Building_Report_July_2012.pdf

Wallerstein, N. B., & Duran, B. (2006). Using community based participatory research to address health disparities. *Health Promotion Practice, 7*(3), 312–323.

Walters, K., Stately, A., Evans-Campbell, T., Simoni, J., Duran, B., Schultz, K., . . . Guerrero, D. (2009). "Indigenist" collaborative research efforts in Native American communities. In A. Stiffman Rubin (Ed.), *The field research survival guide* (pp. 146–173). New York: Oxford University Press.

Walton, R., Zraly, M., & Mugengana, J. P. (2014). Values and validity: Navigating messiness in a community-based research project in Rwanda. *Technical Communication Quarterly, 24*(1), 45–69.

Waterman, H. (1998). Embracing ambiguities and valuing ourselves: Issues of validity in action research. *Journal of Advanced Nursing, 28*(1), 101–105.

Wilson, S. (2008). *Research is ceremony: Indigenous research methods.* Winnipeg, MB, Canada: Fernwood Publishing.

Wolf, D. L. (1996). Situating feminist dilemmas in fieldwork. In D. L. Wolf (Ed.), *Feminist dilemmas in fieldwork* (pp. 1–25). Boulder, CO: Westview Press.

Worthington, C., Chambers, L., Wilson, C., Jackson, R., Tharao, W., Masching, R. (2013). Decolonizing methodologies: Indigenous and African diasporic HIV research. Paper presented at the 2nd International HIV Social Science and Humanities Conference, Paris, France, July 7–10.

Wright, M. T., Roche, B., Von Unger, H., Block, M., & Gardner, B. (2010). A call for an international collaboration on participatory research for health. *Health Promotion International, 25*(1), 115–122.

Index

INDEX

About the Authors

Vera Caine is an associate professor in the Faculty of Nursing at the University of Alberta and a Canadian Institutes of Health Research (CIHR) New Investigator. Caine's research is focused on life-course perspectives in the area of health equity and social justice, particularly to advance health equity for people whose lives are affected by HIV, poverty, social exclusion, and discrimination. Her interest in HIV is longstanding and was first formalized in her early research. Using a visual narrative inquiry approach, Caine worked closely with five urban Aboriginal women, exploring their lives with HIV. Some of the Aboriginal women have stayed in conversation with Caine since then and opened up many questions about the messiness of research, the unfolding of relationships, and how we each are touched by lives and stories, while also exploring issues of differences. In the field of HIV, Caine has engaged in research alongside nurses, women at risk for or living with HIV during their early mothering experience, and most recently alongside children who are at risk for sexual exploitation. Caine also works closely with community agencies. She is a past chair of the board for the Boyle McCauley Health Centre (BMHC), a community health care center in the inner city of Edmonton, and is actively involved in sustaining and developing initiatives that reflect primary health care, value interdisciplinary work, and advocate for a focus on health equity.

Randy Jackson is currently engaged in doctoral studies in the School of Social Work at McMaster University. Recently, he was awarded a predoctoral fellowship leading to an assistant professorship and is now crossappointed in the Department of Health, Aging and Society. He previously completed a BA in social sciences (sociology) from the University of Ottawa (1994) and an MA in sociology from the University of Manitoba (2003). The doctoral program has provided Jackson with an opportunity to further explore the use of Indigenous knowledges in research. The focus of his doctoral research is the experiences and responses to depression among Aboriginal peoples living with HIV. Before his doctoral studies, Jackson was Director of Research, Policy and Programs at the Canadian Aboriginal AIDS Network (CAAN). Originally from Kettle and Stony Point Nation, located in southwestern Ontario, through CAAN Jackson was involved in a number of research projects that engage community and that incorporate Aboriginal values and perspectives (e.g., HIV testing among Aboriginal youth, HIV stigma and use of health services, cultural competence in HIV-related health services, and care, treatment, and support services for Aboriginal people living with HIV).

Renée Masching is a First Nation woman originally from southern Ontario who has dedicated her professional energies to working with Aboriginal peoples in health-related programs. She has worked in addiction programs and in community health education and, for more than 18 years, Masching has been honored to contribute to the Aboriginal HIV and AIDS movement in Canada with dedication and determination. Her contributions include support to community-based HIV/AIDS organizations and working closely with Aboriginal people living with HIV and AIDS; serving as a board member for national organizations; the development of government policy in the Atlantic provinces and federally; and numerous committees and reports. Masching earned BA and MSW degrees from McMaster University with a research award from CIHR. Masching was the executive director of Healing Our Nations, the Atlantic First Nations AIDS Network from 1997 to 2005, and began employment in the fall of 2005 with the Canadian Aboriginal AIDS Network (CAAN) as a community-based research facilitator supporting a community response to HIV and AIDS through research. Presently, Masching is the Director of Research and Policy with CAAN and Principal Knowledge User or Knowledge User on several active research projects. Her research interests are focused on community-based research frameworks, Indigenous knowledge, and community health. Masching is the author/co-author of several peer-reviewed publications and has delivered numerous poster and oral presentations at local, regional, national and international conferences. Masching lives with her husband, sons, and menagerie of pets by the ocean in Mi'kmaq Territory (Nova Scotia).

Judy Mill is a professor emerita at the University of Alberta. She is interested in the social, political, cultural, and economic determinants of HIV infection in vulnerable populations. Her recent research projects have been located in both Canadian and international settings and have focused on the influence of stigma on access to health services by persons with HIV, the involvement of nurses in HIV policy development in sub-Saharan Africa and the Caribbean, and a mentorship intervention for nurses in HIV care. Mill has expertise in qualitative methodologies and community-based research that incorporates opportunities for capacity building in the design. In addition to her public health nursing experience in Canada, Mill has worked for eight years on international health projects in Ghana, Malawi, Rwanda, Zambia, and Zimbabwe.